NUTRITION AND DIET RESEARCH PROGRESS

BREAKFAST

NUTRITION, CONSUMPTION AND HEALTH BENEFITS

NUTRITION AND
DIET RESEARCH PROGRESS

Additional books and e-books in this series can be found on Nova's website under the Series tab.

NUTRITION AND DIET RESEARCH PROGRESS

BREAKFAST

NUTRITION, CONSUMPTION AND HEALTH BENEFITS

PETR MĚCHURA
EDITOR

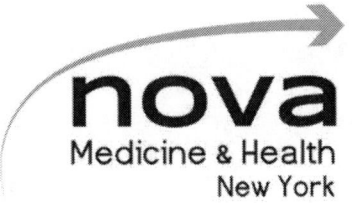

Copyright © 2020 by Nova Science Publishers, Inc.

All rights reserved. No part of this book may be reproduced, stored in a retrieval system or transmitted in any form or by any means: electronic, electrostatic, magnetic, tape, mechanical photocopying, recording or otherwise without the written permission of the Publisher.

We have partnered with Copyright Clearance Center to make it easy for you to obtain permissions to reuse content from this publication. Simply navigate to this publication's page on Nova's website and locate the "Get Permission" button below the title description. This button is linked directly to the title's permission page on copyright.com. Alternatively, you can visit copyright.com and search by title, ISBN, or ISSN.

For further questions about using the service on copyright.com, please contact:
Copyright Clearance Center
Phone: +1-(978) 750-8400   Fax: +1-(978) 750-4470   E-mail: info@copyright.com

NOTICE TO THE READER

The Publisher has taken reasonable care in the preparation of this book, but makes no expressed or implied warranty of any kind and assumes no responsibility for any errors or omissions. No liability is assumed for incidental or consequential damages in connection with or arising out of information contained in this book. The Publisher shall not be liable for any special, consequential, or exemplary damages resulting, in whole or in part, from the readers' use of, or reliance upon, this material. Any parts of this book based on government reports are so indicated and copyright is claimed for those parts to the extent applicable to compilations of such works.

Independent verification should be sought for any data, advice or recommendations contained in this book. In addition, no responsibility is assumed by the Publisher for any injury and/or damage to persons or property arising from any methods, products, instructions, ideas or otherwise contained in this publication.

This publication is designed to provide accurate and authoritative information with regard to the subject matter covered herein. It is sold with the clear understanding that the Publisher is not engaged in rendering legal or any other professional services. If legal or any other expert assistance is required, the services of a competent person should be sought. FROM A DECLARATION OF PARTICIPANTS JOINTLY ADOPTED BY A COMMITTEE OF THE AMERICAN BAR ASSOCIATION AND A COMMITTEE OF PUBLISHERS.

Additional color graphics may be available in the e-book version of this book.

Library of Congress Cataloging-in-Publication Data

Names: Měchura, Petr, editor.
Title: Breakfast : nutrition, consumption and health benefits / [edited by] Petr Měchura.
Description: New York : Nova Science Publishers, [2020] | Series: Nutrition and diet research progress | Includes bibliographical references and index. |
Identifiers: LCCN 2020038887 (print) | LCCN 2020038888 (ebook) | ISBN 9781536185003 (paperback) | ISBN 9781536185966 (adobe pdf)
Subjects: LCSH: Nutrition. | Health. | Breakfasts.
Classification: LCC RA784 .B684 2020 (print) | LCC RA784 (ebook) | DDC 613.2--dc23
LC record available at https://lccn.loc.gov/2020038887
LC ebook record available at https://lccn.loc.gov/2020038888

Published by Nova Science Publishers, Inc. † New York

Contents

Preface		vii
Chapter 1	Nutritional Importance of Breakfast *Janice Ramos de Sousa,* *Rita de Cássia Coelho de Almeida Akutsu,* *Renata Puppin Zandonadi and* *Raquel Braz Assunção Botelho*	1
Chapter 2	Potential Benefits of Choosing Plant-Based Meals for Breakfast *Shila Minari Hargreaves,* *Raquel Braz Assunção Botelho* *and Renata Puppin Zandonadi*	33
Chapter 3	Gluten-Containing Products in Breakfast and Their Substitutes in Gluten-Related Disorders *Renata Puppin Zandonadi and* *Raquel Braz Assunção Botelho*	59
Chapter 4	Gluten-Free Breakfast in Brazilian Public Schools: The Menu Adequacy to the National Program *Iris Veleci da Silva Santos, Ana Luisa Falcomer,* *Priscila Farage and Renata Puppin Zandonadi*	83

Chapter 5	Dairy Products in Breakfast and Their Substitutes in the Milk Restriction Diet *Priscila Farage, Luana Rincon, Renata Puppin Zandonadi and Raquel Braz Assunção Botelho*	**103**
Index		**123**

PREFACE

Despite being one of the most important meals of the day, breakfast is also the most neglected meal of the day, and this practice increases progressively with age because of lack of time, organization, or individual's preference.

Breakfast: Nutrition, Consumption and Health Benefits discusses how a breakfast based on fruits, vegetables, and whole grains can lead to a more favorable lipid profile, contributing to diabetes prevention and control without the harmful effects of eating sugary industrialized foods.

The authors advocate that evaluation of breakfast gluten-containing products and their counterparts without gluten is important for people with gluten-related disorders.

Additionally, they discuss how visibility of the difficulties faced in the implementation of special menus for children with celiac disease in Brazilian public schools can contribute to making the Human Right to Adequate Food a reality for this group.

In closing, the authors assess the importance of finding viable options with sensory and nutritional quality that can be part of the diet of individuals who restrict milk.

Chapter 1 - Despite being one of the most important meals of the day, breakfast is also the most neglected meal of the day, and this practice increases progressively with age because of lack of time, organization, or individual's preference. Little attention is given to breakfast's nutritional composition, mainly when carried out of home. The first meal of the day should be before or at the beginning of the daily activities with an energy value that ranges from 15 to 25% of the total energetic needs according to different studies. Researchers relate the frequent consumption of breakfast to the low risk of overweight and obesity. Some of the benefits of having this meal are satiety, less energy daily intake, better glycemic control, lower risk of weight gain, and comorbidities related to weight. The nutritional quality of breakfast should be studied and discussed to evaluate the associations to health benefits. There is a strong cultural component related to breakfast that influences the food choices, and consequently, the nutritional quality. Some authors state that breakfast should include three basic food groups, dairy, cereals, and fruits because they are closely related to nutritional status.

Chapter 2 - Evidence shows that eating breakfast has positive effects on health, mainly due to better food intake during the day and hormonal profile. However, the nutritional quality of the meal must be taken into account to guarantee these health benefits. Over the last years, health professionals, studies, and media have put effort into encouraging a reduction of refined carbohydrates intake (sugary cereals, white bread, and sugary beverages such as artificial juices or milk chocolate), considering a traditional western diet breakfast. Despite a potential positive effect of reducing sugar and refined foods intake in health, breakfast recommendations have shifted towards more animal-based meals, which include eggs, bacon, cheese, and even coffee with butter (bulletproof coffee). In the short-term, these foods might indeed bring some benefits, such as lower ghrelin levels (resulting in more satiety) and lower post-prandial glycemic peaks. On the other hand, a single high saturated fat meal or high animal protein meal can increase inflammatory markers over the following hours and the risk of non-communicable diseases and mortality, leading to worse gut microbiome profile. A fiber plant-based meal can have better effects on health, equally contributing to satiety and, at the same time, helping to reduce inflammatory markers and improve microbiome health. A breakfast based on fruits, vegetables, and whole grains, such as oatmeal or whole-grain bread, can lead to a more favorable lipid profile, contributing to diabetes and overweight prevention and control, without the harmful effects of eating sugary industrialized foods. It is essential to stimulate the consumption of breakfast and a higher intake of calories during the morning period compared to night time. However, the use of whole-foods plant-based breakfast should be encouraged instead of an animal-based meal to guarantee long-term health benefits.

Chapter 3 - The adverse reactions to gluten-containing products are increasing worldwide. Gluten-related disorders (GRD) include celiac disease, non-celiac gluten sensitivity, gluten ataxia, gluten, or wheat allergy, among others, reaching almost 10% of the worldwide population following the gluten-free diet (GFD). Breakfast is one of the meals that present a high consumption of gluten-containing foods (bread, cake, pancake, waffle, cereals, cookies, crackers, etc.). Breakfast is described as one of the most important meals of the day, generally consumed before going to work and reaching close to 20% of the nutritional recommendations. Therefore, it is a challenge to substitute gluten-containing products in breakfast due to the population's habit of consumption, the lack of gluten-free with nutritional, sensory, and technological quality, the cost of the substitutes, among others. In this context, the evaluation of breakfast gluten-containing products and their counterparts without gluten is important to help people with GRD to adequate their diet and to reduce the psychological burden of GFD.

Chapter 4 - In Brazil, the right to food was included as a fundamental right in the Federal Constitution. Among the Brazilian initiatives that contribute to guaranteeing the Human Right to Adequate Food (HRAF/*DHAA*) is the National School Food Program (NSFP/*PNAE*). Since 2014, offering special menus for children with food restrictions has become mandatory, as in cases of children with gluten-related disorders (GRD). In Brazilian public schools, GRD individuals commonly report that there are not substitutes for the gluten-containing foods offered. In some cases, the meal offered at school represents the main meal for low-income children living in a situation of food scarcity at home. Moreover, when alternative gluten-free food is provided, itis not safe for the students due to issues such as gluten cross-contamination. Therefore, the visibility of the difficulties faced in the implementation of special menus for children with celiac disease in Brazilian public schools can contribute to making the Human Right to Adequate Food a reality for this group.

Chapter 5 - Breakfast is considered the most important meal of the day. Breakfast options vary a lot worldwide according to cultural feeding habits in different populations. However, milk and its derived products are a common food choice across countries. Milk as a drink is usually consumed with coffee or pure, or it might be combined with cereals in a bowl. Other alternatives include milk derivatives such as yogurt and curd, which may be ingested pure, served with fruits and bread, and used to prepare smoothies. Different types of cheese are also commonly present in the population breakfast. Additionally, there are many other food options, which include milk or other milk ingredients in their recipes. The cultural presence of milk in the diet and its extensive use in the food industry, in general, make it complicated for people who need to adopt a milk-free diet. Some conditions, such as cow's milk allergy and lactose intolerance, demand a restriction of milk in the diet. Vegetarian individuals also restrict milk as a lifestyle choice. In these cases, non-dairy derived substitute products may appear in the individual's diet. However, cow's milk and its derivatives display sensorial features appreciated by the population and essential nutritional characteristics, such as its high protein and calcium content. Therefore, it is important to find viable options with sensory and nutritional quality that can be part of the diet of individuals who restrict milk.

In: Breakfast
Editor: Petr Měchura

ISBN: 978-1-53618-500-3
© 2020 Nova Science Publishers, Inc.

Chapter 1

NUTRITIONAL IMPORTANCE OF BREAKFAST

Janice Ramos de Sousa,
Rita de Cássia Coelho de Almeida Akutsu,
Renata Puppin Zandonadi
and Raquel Braz Assunção Botelho[*]
Department of Nutrition, University of Brasília, Brasília, DF, Brazil

ABSTRACT

Despite being one of the most important meals of the day, breakfast is also the most neglected meal of the day, and this practice increases progressively with age because of lack of time, organization, or individual's preference. Little attention is given to breakfast's nutritional composition, mainly when carried out of home. The first meal of the day should be before or at the beginning of the daily activities with an energy value that ranges from 15 to 25% of the total energetic needs according to different studies. Researchers relate the frequent consumption of breakfast to the low risk of overweight and obesity. Some of the benefits of having this meal are satiety, less energy daily intake, better glycemic control, lower risk of weight gain, and comorbidities related to weight. The

---

[*] Corresponding Author's E-mail: raquelbabotelho@gmail.com.

nutritional quality of breakfast should be studied and discussed to evaluate the associations to health benefits. There is a strong cultural component related to breakfast that influences the food choices, and consequently, the nutritional quality. Some authors state that breakfast should include three basic food groups, dairy, cereals, and fruits because they are closely related to nutritional status.

Keywords: nutrients, breakfast, composition, food choices

INTRODUCTION

Studies have been seeking to identify consumption in specific populations (such as adolescents, children, or adults) and different cultures (Díaz-Torrente and Quintiliano-Scarpelli 2020; Melo et al. 2020; Baltar et al. 2018; Zakrzewski-Fruer et al. 2017; Monteiro et al. 2017b). They pointed out some trends regarding the eating behavior of people in industrialized societies or not, such as the search for diversity, the appreciation of food outside the home, the increase in consumption of industrialized foods, the replacement of meals and traditional preparations with snacks with a high concentration of energy, fat, sugar and sodium (Ruiz et al. 2018; Drewnowski, Rehm, and Vieux 2018; Gibney, Barr, Bellisle, Drewnowski, Fagt, Hopkins, et al. 2018; Bellisle et al. 2018; Scheen and Van Gaal 2014; Gibney, Barr, Bellisle, Drewnowski, Fagt, Livingstone, et al. 2018; A. M. Souza et al. 2013; Baltar et al. 2018; Díaz-Torrente and Quintiliano-Scarpelli 2020).

These situations provide the disruption of meals, where breakfast (BF) is the most neglected meal (Affinita et al. 2013a; Freitas, Mendonça, and Lopes 2013; Hallström et al. 2011; Huang et al. 2016; Nurul-Fadhilah et al. 2013; Trancoso, Cavalli, and Proença 2010; Jomori, Proença, and Calvo 2008; R. P. C. Proença 2010; Zakrzewski-Fruer et al. 2017) contrasting the findings that showed that regular consumption of BF could lower Body Mass Index-BMI (Williams 2014; Szajewska and Ruszczyński 2010), cardiovascular risk (di Giuseppe et al. 2012; Iqbal et al. 2017; Kubota et al. 2016; Hallström et al. 2013), and improve cognitive function (Hoyland, Dye, and Lawton 2009) compared to individuals who skip BF. Some studies stated that it is not only consumption or suppression of eating that is most important but the quality of what is consumed (Monteiro et al. 2017b; Baltar et al. 2018; Drewnowski, Rehm, and Vieux 2018). Therefore, it is a consensus that the presence and quality of BF are essential for maintaining health and preventing diseases (Cardoso et al. 2009; Yoo et al. 2014; Freitas, Mendonça, and Lopes 2013; Baltar et al. 2018), showing the importance of the knowledge about the nutritional quality of the BF. Considering that the quality of food or meals must be a human-centered process, it can be perceived from a variety of perspectives, such as nutritional, sensory, hygienic-sanitary, service, regulatory, symbolic, and the social (R. P. da C. Proença et al. 2005). The quality approach focus of this chapter will be the nutritional one, which concerns the characteristics and benefits of nutrients found in foods consumed in BF.

There is evidence to suggest that adequate daily consumption of BF is associated with the choice of foods richer in nutrients, such as fruits, vegetables, dairy products, and whole-grains (Fagt et al. 2018; Enes and Slater 2010; Nurul-Fadhilah et al. 2013). Thus, BF represents an opportunity for the consumption of foods rich in proteins, calcium, vitamins, minerals, and fibers that go beyond the issue of consumption or suppression (Höfelmann and Momm 2014; Gibney, Barr, Bellisle, Drewnowski, Fagt, Hopkins, et al. 2018; Ruiz et al. 2018). Despite the globalization, the countries present differences in the BF constitution, and as a consequence in the nutritional composition. Spence (2017) discusses that beyond cultural differences in BF, there are other psycho-physiological reasons that lead consumers to different foods. The author also states that there are a variety of reasons for consedering BF the most important meal of the day.

THE ENERGY CONTRIBUTION OF BREAKFAST IN ENERGY CONSUMPTION

The percentage of BF energy contribution in daily energy consumption is information that still differs between the authors. According to Pereira et al. (M. A. Pereira et al. 2011), BF should represent an energy level between 20 and 35% of the total daily consumed calories. For other authors, the BF must have an energy content that meets 20-25% of the overall daily energy needs (Monteagudo et al. 2013; Fernández Morales et al. 2011; van den Boom et al. 2006). For Marangoni et al. (Marangoni et al. 2009), regular consumption of BF should provide 15 to 20% of the daily caloric intake. Trancoso, Cavalli e Proença (Trancoso, Cavalli, and Proença 2010) are more categorical when informing that the Brazilian recommendation is that the BF guarantees, on average, 25% of the total energy consumed during the day, varying from 15 to 35% of the total daily caloric intake. In this sense, BF would represent an average consumption of 500 kcal in a daily diet of 2000 kcal.

According to Bispo (Bispo, and Roncada 2006), in a study whose objective was to trace the food profile of the BF of professors from the University of Brasilia, a percentage energy contribution from BF varied from 25% to 36%. de Sousa, Botelho, Akutsu, & Zandonadi (2019) evaluated BF consumption in low-income Brazilians, and the mean energy intake was 340.5 kcal, representing 17% in a 2000 kcal diet.

The reflection of the energy contribution of BF in the total daily caloric value is a matter of debate. There are currently two strands of knowledge, one of which believes that omitting BF (Nicklas et al. 1998) or performing a high-calorie BF does not induce energy compensation for absent or extra calories in later meals. The other side argues that a BF with a higher energy contribution is associated with lower daily energy consumption, through less efficiency in the use of energy.

This double conception about the energy participation of BF in the total daily caloric value is what motivated the research by Schusdziarra et al. (Schusdziarra et al. 2011). These authors analyzed the intra-individual energy consumption of a group of 280 obese and 100 individuals with adequate weight. Data were analyzed considering the energy consumption in the BF and the proportion of the contribution of that meal in the total energy intake. The study concluded that the reduction in BF energy consumption is associated with a lower total daily intake. Thus, suppression of BF can be useful to decrease daily intake and improve energy balance during the treatment of obesity (Schusdziarra et al. 2011).

It is important to emphasize that diets with lower energy density are associated with a better quality of food in the BF, especially concerning the consumption of cereals and fruits (Affinita et al. 2013b).

NUTRITIONAL CONTRIBUTION FROM BREAKFAST

The type of food consumed in the BF is critical because it defines different patterns of nutrient intake (Min et al. 2012; Monteiro et al. 2017a; Hassan et al. 2018; Baltar et al. 2018), which vary according to the culture (di Giuseppe et al. 2012; Baltar et al. 2018; Melo et al. 2020; Kubota et al. 2016; Hassan et al. 2018). The Japanese and Korean BF, for example, consists of fish, soy, eggs, algae, tofu, and vegetables, all of which are rich in protein, vitamins, minerals and low in fat, very different from the western BF, which consists of bread, eggs, dairy products, cereals and meats (Melby and Takeda 2014; Höfelmann and Momm 2014). The population of the United States generally consumes bread, eggs, fruit, ready-to-eat cereal and milk, coffee, juice, and soft drinks (Deshmukh-Taskar et al. 2013). The consumption of vegetables, sources of dietary fiber, folate, zinc, iron, and magnesium, in BF is more frequent among Hispanic Americans (O'Neil et al. 2014).

In Brazil, as it is a country of continental dimension and very culturally diverse, there is a very different pattern of consumption and quality of food in the BF between the Brazilian regions (de Sousa et al. 2019; Carrijo et al. 2018; Ginani et al. 2010). Baltar et al. (Baltar et al. 2018) studied the relationship between BMI, suppressing breakfast, and breakfast patterns in Brazilian adults. Data from 21,003 Brazilian adults (20 and 59 years) from the National Diet Survey showed that suppressing breakfast was not associated with BMI in this population. They also showed that BF composed of cold meats, milk, cheese, coffee, tea, and bread was inversely associated with BMI. BF with meats, corn-foods, eggs, tubers, roots, potatoes, dairy products, snacks, crackers, fruit juices, soy-based drinks were positively associated with BMI.

Also, in Brazil, Hassan et al. (Hassan et al. 2018) performed a cohort-study to analyze changes in the frequency and consumption of 809 adolescents. The authors concluded that overweight/obese adolescents were more likely to have an irregular BF at the beginning than those who were not overweight/obese. After three years, individuals with overweight/obesity had a higher risk of low consumption of fruits and of skipping breakfast.

In Australia, Fayet-Moore et al. (Fayet-Moore et al. 2017) studied the BF of 2821 adolescents aged 2 to 18 years. Participants were classified as breakfast cereal consumers (minimally pre-sweetened (MPS) or pre-sweetened (PS), non-cereal breakfast consumers, or breakfast skippers. Foods consumed for breakfast, foods added to the cereal bowl, and the impact of BF choice on daily nutrient intake and anthropometric measures were determined. Although only 9% of the children skipped breakfast, 61% of the skippers were aged 14–18 years. Among BF consumers, 49% had breakfast cereal, and 62% of these exclusively consumed MPS cereal. Breakfast skippers had a higher saturated fat intake than breakfast cereal consumers, and lower intakes of dietary fibre and most micronutrients ($p < 0.001$). Compared with non-cereal breakfast consumers, breakfast cereal consumers had similar added and free sugars intakes, lower sodium, and higher total sugars, carbohydrate, dietary fibre, and almost all other micronutrients ($p < 0.001$). The only difference in nutrient intakes between MPS and PS cereal consumers was higher folate among PS consumers. No associations between anthropometric measures and BF or breakfast cereal choice were found (Fayet-Moore et al. 2017).

In Spain, there was a study to nutritionally analyze the consumption of BF and lunch with 740 university students, and the result showed that the percentage of vitamin and mineral intake was significantly higher in BF than that consumed at lunch (Durá Travé 2013). The most consumed food groups in the BF of the participants in this study were dairy products (92.6%), cereals (58.8%) and the group of sweet sweets, cakes and bakery products (57.9%), as marmalades, products with chocolates, cookies, croissants, muffins, etc. The result of the Spanish study clearly shows the cultural influence on the eating habits of consuming sweet foods in the first meal of the day (Durá Travé 2013).

Souza et al. (F. M. Souza et al. 2007) studied 400 adult patients from a dietitian's office in the southern part of the city of São Paulo, Brazil. They applied a 24-hour food record, which was limited to the homemade quantities of food and drinks reported by patients during breakfast. The authors defined BF as any drink or food ingested in the meal called by the patient as BF. Individuals who did not eat or drink, excluding water, were categorized as "without breakfast"(F. M. Souza et al. 2007).

The analysis of food consumption in this study (F. M. Souza et al. 2007) showed that the most consumed food categories were fats and sweets (margarine, butter, powdered chocolate, sugar, ready-to-drink chocolate, industrialized juices, chocolate, pizza, and soft drinks); milk and dairy products (skimmed, semi-skimmed or whole milk, skimmed or whole yogurt, cheeses, creamy cheese, fermented milk, soy milk); meats and eggs (omelet, tuna, salami, beef); fruits and vegetables (orange, carrot, papaya, mango, natural juices, and dried fruits); cereals (granola, oats, corn flakes and cereal bars); bread (white, wholegrain, soft bread, cracker, toast, corn, cheese bread, cornmeal, potato bread, croissant); sweet cakes and cookies (stuffed cookies, panettone, and cakes); and drinks (tea, coffee, cappuccino) (F. M. Souza et al. 2007).

In Iran, Azadbakht et al. (Azadbakht et al. 2013) assessed the association between BF consumption and food quality, using the Healthy Eating Index, the Food Diversity Score, and anthropometric measures. They evaluated 411 university adult females (18 and 29 years old) and showed that the consumption of BF was associated with a higher quality of the diet and lower values of BMI. Corroborating these findings, Soares and Ping-Delfos (Soares and Chan She Ping-Delfos 2008) affirm that there is an assumption among researchers on the topic, suggesting that the nutritional composition of the first meal of the day may have implications for the energy metabolism of the rest of the day.

Pedersen et al. (Pedersen et al. 2012) investigated the association between irregular consumption of BF and the consumption of fruits and vegetables in 3,913 adolescents in Denmark. The results showed that irregular BF was associated with a low frequency of consumption of fruits and vegetables, and gender and age can play a role in modifying this behavior. These results highlight the importance of encouraging daily BF among adolescents since the tendency is to maintain this behavior in adulthood.

Herrera (Herrera 2007) studied 121 Venezuelan students with higher education to know the consumption of basic food groups according to several variables, including gender. The results of the study, which lasted one year, showed an evident scarcity in the intake of vegetables and fruits, mainly in BF and at dinner. Male students ate fewer vegetables and fruits for lunch and dinner, while women ate less of these foods in BF. In short, fruit consumption proved to be deficient in BF, mainly among females.

Drewnowski, Rehm e Vieux (Drewnowski, Rehm, and Vieux 2018) analyzed from the first reported day of the National Health and Examination Survey (NHANES) 2011-2014 in the United States (n = 14,488) BF associated with better quality diets. The Diet Quality measures were the Nutrient Rich Food Index (NRF9.3) and the USDA Healthy Food Index 2015 (IES 2015). The results showed that four out of five NHANES participants had BF. BF provided 19-22% of the energy of the diet and more than 20% of the daily intake of B vitamins, vitamins A and D, folate, calcium, iron, potassium, and magnesium. Finally, the authors conclude that BF patterns that favored fruits, whole grains, and dairy products were associated with healthier diets.

Gibney et al. (Gibney, Barr, Bellisle, Drewnowski, Fagt, Hopkins, et al. 2018) established nutritional recommendations for a balanced BF using a standardized analysis of national nutrition surveys in Canada, Denmark, France, Spain, the United Kingdom, and the USA. In all countries, the frequency of BF consumption by age was high and U-shaped, with children and the elderly with a higher rate of BF consumption. BF contributed to 16% to 21% of the daily energy intake. In all countries, BF was a meal providing more carbohydrates (including sugars), thiamine, riboflavin, folate, calcium, potassium, and magnesium and less vitamin A, fats, and sodium concerning their contribution for the daily intake of nutrients.

Sievert et al. (Sievert et al. 2019) performed a systematic review with meta-analysis to examine the effect of BF on weight or energy intake. They were searched by randomized clinical trials published between January 1990 and January 2018. The results showed that of the 13 included trials, seven examined the effect of BF consumption on weight change, and 10 examined the impact on energy intake. A meta-analysis of the results found a small difference in weight, favoring participants who did not consume BF (mean difference of 0.44 kg, 95% confidence interval from 0.07 to 0.82). However, there was some inconsistency in the test results. Participants who consumed BF had a higher total daily energy intake than those who suppressed breakfast (mean difference 259.79 kcal/day)(Sievert et al. 2019). The authors point out that all included studies had a high or unclear risk of bias in at least one domain and had only short-term follow-up (average period of seven weeks for weight, two weeks for energy intake). As the quality of the included studies was mainly low, the results should be interpreted with caution (Sievert et al. 2019). Therefore, the study's analysis suggests that adding BF may not be a good strategy for weight loss, regardless of the established habit for BF.

In another systematic review with meta-analysis with ten studies, Brown et al. (Brown et al. 2017) concluded that there seems to be no significant effect between consuming or suppressing breakfast on anthropometric measures related to obesity.

Even though there is a diversity of foods consumed worldwide, the authors Travé (Durá Travé 2013) and O'Neil et al. (O'Neil et al. 2014) stated that BF must include at least three primary groups: dairy, cereals, and fruits, as the type of food consumed in BF that have specific effects on nutritional status. For example, eating cereals or bread in the BF has been associated with a significantly lower BMI when compared to those who omitted the BF or consumed meat and/or eggs in this meal (Cho et al. 2003).

Worldwide, the most abundant foods in essential micronutrients consumed in BF are milk and dairy products. For this reason, they should always be present on the BF menu and should preferably be combined with complex carbohydrates as an energy source. Also, milk is a source of high-quality nutritional protein and an essential source of calcium, phosphorus, and essential amino acids (Affinita et al. 2013b; Bonjour et al. 2013). However, there is a tendency to substitute these foods since cow's milk protein is the most frequent cause of food allergies and intolerances. (Laissa et al. 2013).

One of the nutrients considered essential in a balanced BF is fiber, supplied mainly by fruits, vegetables, and whole grains. It acts positively on glucose metabolism and insulin response (Marangoni et al. 2009), reducing the risk of developing type 2 diabetes and being overweight. Pedersen et al. (Pedersen et al. 2012) also state that diets rich in fruits and vegetables reduce the risk of cardiovascular disease and some types of cancer.

Calcium is an essential nutrient in several biological functions, such as muscle contraction, mitosis, blood clotting, the transmission of nervous or synaptic impulse, and bone structure. Thus, calcium intake can prevent diseases such as osteoporosis, high blood pressure, colon cancer, and obesity (Ahmed et al. 2012). Increased calcium intake can reduce body fat (G. A. P. Pereira et al. 2009) since it influences the activity of enzymes involved in fat synthesis and lipolysis (Soares and Chan She Ping-Delfos 2008).

Galas, Augustyniak e Sochacka-Tatara (Galas, Augustyniak, and Sochacka-Tatara 2013) conducted a study to assess the effect of high levels of calcium intake and the risk of developing colorectal cancer. The study's result confirmed the protective effect of higher doses of calcium in the diet against the risk of colon cancer. The results support the evidence for the potential advantage of an increase in food consumption at the same meal that are sources of calcium and fiber.

The only source of calcium available to the human body is that from the diet, it is essential to ensure a minimum intake of the mineral to allow bone growth and maintenance (Bueno and Czepielewski 2008). O'Neil et al. (O'Neil et al. 2014) suggest that the appropriate intake of calcium in the BF is between 200 and 300 mg. This amount of calcium intake in BF is because this mineral is lost daily by the body in considerable quantities. If this loss is not compensated by a corresponding amount, consumed via food, the body breaks down bone structure units to provide calcium for circulation (Bedani and Rossi 2005). In Brasil, studies (Leal et al. 2010; Triches and Giugliani 2005; Vieira, Del Ciampo, and Del Ciampo 2014) have focused on the habit of having BF and its relationship with calcium intake in children and adolescents, but studies with adults are rare.

A study that evaluated the association of obesity with dietary practices in 573 students from Rio Grande do Sul/Brazil found that the habit of not taking BF is significantly associated with low milk consumption and obesity (Triches and Giugliani 2005). This data shows that the suppression of this meal negatively affects the supply of proteins and minerals, such as calcium, which should be supplied by the consumption of foods that make up the diet of children, adolescents, and adults.

Assessing the habits and food consumption of 130 adolescents from two public schools in Ribeirão Preto/Brazil, the authors (Vieira, Del Ciampo, and Del Ciampo 2014) hypothesized that the suppression of BF, which in this case was 14%, as well as the morning (54.8%) and afternoon (16.1%) snacks, helped in the low intake of fruits and milk and dairy, contributing to the low consumption of fibers, vitamins, and minerals, including calcium.

Leal et al. (Leal et al. 2010) conducted a study with 228 adolescents in the State of São Paulo, Brazil, whose objective was to assess food consumption and the pattern of meals of adolescents. The results indicated that 96% of the females and 90% of the males had calcium intake below the recommendation. Low calcium consumption showed a direct correlation with 21% suppression of BF among adolescents, with this rate being higher among girls (29%) compared to boys (13%), with a positive association between the female gender and not having this meal (Leal et al. 2010).

In cases of substitution of milk for drinks with low calcium content, such as tea, coffee, juices, plant-based milk, and soft drinks, calcium consumption is directly affected. In cases of substitution of milk for tea, it is important to emphasize that the tannins from tea, can form insoluble complexes with calcium, reducing its absorption. However, these components seem to affect calcium absorption only when the diet is not balanced (G. A. P. Pereira et al. 2009). Plant-based or non-dairy milk alternative is the most frequent product to substitute milk since cow milk allergy, lactose intolerance, and preference to vegan diets influences consumers on choosing cow milk alternatives. However, the majority of milk alternatives lack nutritional balance compared to cow milk, but they may contain functional components with health-promoting properties (Sethi, Tyagi, and Anurag 2016). Some authors achieved plant-based milk with calcium and protein content, similar to cows' milk (Pineli et al. 2015; Arruda Daguer Damasceno, Assunção Botelho, and Rodrigues de Alencar 2020). This theme is explored in another chapter of this book.

Frequent substitution of milk for coffee is also not adequate due to the harmful effect of caffeine on bone mineral density (Luz 2007). The consumption of caffeine with calcium absorption has been much discussed, but the moderate use of this substance does not harm bone health. However, excessive doses of caffeine can result in increased calcium excretion, thus increasing the risk of osteoporosis. The effects of caffeine on bone tissue have been correlated with increased calciuria and decreased efficiency of intestinal calcium absorption. These mechanisms can promote a negative balance in calcium metabolism, thus harming bone metabolism and leading to a significantly more significant reduction in bone mass. (Harter et al. 2013). Higdon and Frei (Higdon and Frei 2006) claim that a balanced diet with moderate consumption of coffee, limited to three cups (equivalent to 710 ml) per day (300 mg/day of caffeine), is not harmful to calcium absorption.

The exchange of milk to soft drinks is even more harmful to health, as these are drinks of low nutritional quality. The colas-based drinks have a more significant aggravating factor, as they contain caffeine and phosphoric acid, which can negatively affect the bioavailability of calcium. This effect happens because of the generation of acidic charge in the body caused by the phosphoric acid used as an acidulant in these drinks (Morais and Burgos 2007). This trend (observed in children, adolescents, and young adults) reflects negatively on bone health in two ways: first, the availability of calcium in the growth and development phases can be compromised; second, the substances contained in soft drinks prevent the fixation of calcium in the bone matrix (Brasil. Ministério da Saúde. 2008).

Vitamin D is another nutrient intrinsically related to the consumption of BF because it is closely connected to the metabolism of calcium in the body. When the consumption of vitamin D source foods is insufficient, it can interfere with calcium absorption (Maeda et al. 2014; Morais and Burgos 2007).

Another factor that can influence the bioavailability of calcium is sodium since the high intake of this nutrient causes an increase in renal calcium excretion (Morais and Burgos 2007; G. A. P. Pereira et al. 2009). Pereira et al. (G. A. P. Pereira et al. 2009) consider that increasing calcium intake attenuates salt sensitivity and reduces blood pressure, especially in hypertensive individuals, highlighting the importance of consuming food sources of calcium in BF.

Sodium has been linked to the BF meal worldwide, as bread is a significant contributor to the high intake of this mineral, as it brings a high concentration of it in its composition (Bolhuis et al. 2011). In the analysis of a simple meal of BF composed of bread with butter/margarine and coffee with milk, one of the primary nutrients worthy of concern is the possible excess of sodium intake, as it is a risk factor for the development of cardiovascular diseases. Milk is a natural source of sodium, and generally, the healthy population consumes butter/margarine with salt, and most bread receives salt in its recipe. Therefore, the consumption of this mineral can easily exceed the recommended average daily amount, after considering its consumption at all meals of the day.

Thus, high sodium intake at all meals and even in BF, due to the consumption of bread, is directly related to high blood pressure and an increased risk factor for cardiovascular diseases, the leading cause of mortality in the world. Increasing evidence suggests that high sodium intake is also related to kidney disease and has been identified as a major cause of stomach cancer. The consumption of foods such as sausages and some cheeses also influences sodium intake. It should receive extra attention regarding its presence on the daily menu, especially for people with such pathologies (Ignácio et al. 2013; Sarno et al. 2009; Bolhuis et al. 2011; Brasil. Ministério da Saúde. 2008).

According to WHO (World Health Organization (WHO) 2011), the nutritional need for sodium for humans is 500 milligrams, which corresponds to about 1.2 grams of sodium chloride (table salt). WHO also defined that the maximum amount considered healthy for daily food intake, being 5g of sodium chloride or table salt (which corresponds to 2g sodium). Despite the fact of these limits for sodium consumption, the average consumption of the Brazilian population corresponds approximately to twice that recommended (Brasil 2011; Zandonadi et al. 2014). A recent systematic review and meta-analysis (Carrillo-Larco and Bernabe-Ortiz 2020) of sodium consumption estimated sodium consumption of 4.13 g/day (10.49 g/day of salt) in Latin America and the Caribbean. A study assessed the mean level of global sodium intake about 3.95 g per day ranging from 2.18 to 5.51 g per day (Mozaffarian et al. 2014). In this sense, globally, 1.65 million annual deaths from cardiovascular causes were attributed to high sodium intake above the reference level (Mozaffarian et al. 2014).

It is interesting to note that the products with the highest sodium content are not always the ones that most contribute to the intake of this nutrient. For example, instant noodles are a product with high sodium content. Still, they do not participate in people's daily diets like bread, which is consumed more times a day, becoming a permanent source of sodium (Idec 2015).

Due to its high sodium content and its essential role in daily consumption, bread is a significant contributor to sodium intake in the diet of many countries (Meneton et al. 2009; Strazzullo et al. 2012; Bolhuis et al. 2011). Gibson and Ashwell (Gibson and Ashwell 2011) examined dietary patterns among British adults and associations of sodium with macronutrient intake, and bread was the most significant contributor to total sodium intake, accounting for 22% of sodium intake for men and 21% for women.

Souza et al. (de Moura Souza et al. 2013) analyzed data from one of the Brazilian Budget Survey modules 2008-2009, considering individuals of both sexes. Data analysis showed that salt bread was one of the five most consumed foods (63%) and that its availability within the household corresponds to 6% of the total calories. From the analysis carried out by the authors, it was estimated that more than 70% of the Brazilian population consumed excess sodium (more than 2,000 mg a day) and that more than 90% of adults and adolescents aged 14 to 18 in urban areas exceed this daily limit.

Concern similar to sodium should be given to the intake of saturated fats, especially trans-hydrogenated fatty acids, present in margarine, crackers, cookies, ice cream, chips, pastries and bakery products consumed in BF, requiring attention due to its unfavorable effects on human health (Marangoni et al. 2009). They have been negatively associated with cardiovascular diseases, chronic degenerative diseases, intrauterine growth, obesity, and inflammatory diseases. (Ansorena et al. 2013; Benatar and Stewart 2014; Wang et al. 2013).

Trans fatty acids are triglycerides that contain unsaturated fatty acids with one or more trans double bonds, expressed as free fatty acids (Araújo et al. 2014). In other words, trans fatty acids are vegetable oils, therefore liquid, which undergo a partial hydrogenation process capable of converting liquid oils into pasty substances. They are rarely found in their natural state but are present in the milk and meat of ruminant animals. One of the primary sources of trans fatty acids in the diet comes from partially hydrogenated vegetable oil used in the processing of some products widely consumed in the typical western diet (Bertolino et al. 2006; Aued-Pimentel et al. 2009; Castro et al. 2009; Cortés et al. 2013).

Trans fatty acids are neither essential nor offer health benefits. For this reason, the Dietary Reference Intakes (DRI), which is a nutritional recommendation system considered in almost all countries of the world, do not indicate recommendations for consumption or maximum tolerated value for this type of fat (Da Costa Proença and Silveira 2012).

Because of the importance of the theme, WHO launched the Global Strategy for the Promotion of Healthy Eating, Physical Activity, and Health, establishing, among other aspects, the elimination of the consumption of trans fatty acids as a goal. WHO demonstrated concern over the intake of trans fats by recommending a review of its tolerable limit, which was up to 1% of daily energy consumption, and which is still in force in many countries (Da Costa Proença and Silveira 2012).

Nestel (Nestel 2014) considers that coordinated actions between nutritionists, food regulators and the food industry to reduce or eliminate the harmful effects of trans fatty acids in foods are one of the few success stories in the area of nutrition.

The interest and joint effort of different actors in different countries, governments, industries, and society is an extremely commendable action in reducing the amount of trans fat available in the market. In order to better serve the satisfaction of taste and practicality in the food, the food industry has invested heavily in the offer of new products and the insertion of trans fat in the preparation of various foodstuffs, mainly in bakery and confectionery products.

It is observed that, as in every meal, it is essential to pay attention to the type of food to be consumed in the BF, as each food group offers a particular variety of essential nutrients. The essence of a balanced diet is to harmonize the presence of all food groups to guarantee the necessary constituents for the promotion and maintenance of human health.

Final Considerations

BF consumption is vital for many reasons, according to different studies presented in this chapter. Serious health consequences can emerge from the lack of something to eat at the beginning of the day, such as heart disease, obesity, and cognitive performance. However, many studies did not relate suppression or not of BF with anthropometric measures.

BF energy contribution varies among countries and studies, and there is not a consensus on the percentage of daily energy intake. The literature presents from 15% to 35% the contribution of BF during the day. Food choices and nutrients intake also vary because of different cultures and habits, ranging from bread, cereals, milk, and fruits to fish, meat, legumes, and fermented products. It is not possible to define the correct choice of foods for BF. Still, researchers are showing more attention is necessary for the reduction of sodium, trans-fatty acids, and sugar intake at the first meal of the day.

References

Affinita, Antonio, Loredana Catalani, Giovanna Cecchetto, Gianfranco De Lorenzo, Dario Dilillo, Giorgio Donegani, Lucia Fransos, et al. 2013a.

"Breakfast: A Multidisciplinary Approach." *Italian Journal of Pediatrics* 39 (1): 44. https://doi.org/10.1186/1824-7288-39-44.

———. 2013b. "Breakfast: A Multidisciplinary Approach." *Italian Journal of Pediatrics*. BioMed Central. https://doi.org/10.1186/1824-7288-39-44.

Ahmed, Anwaar, Faqir Muhammad Anjum, Muhammad Atif Randhawa, Umar Farooq, Saeed Akhtar, and Muhammad Tauseef Sultan. 2012. "Effect of Multiple Fortification on the Bioavailability of Minerals in Wheat Meal Bread." *Journal of Food Science and Technology* 49 (6): 737. https://doi.org/10.1007/S13197-010-0224-9.

Ansorena, Diana, Andrea Echarte, Rebeca Ollé, and Iciar Astiasarán. 2013. "2012: No Trans Fatty Acids in Spanish Bakery Products." *Food Chemistry* 138 (1): 422–29. https://doi.org/10.1016/j.foodchem.2012.10.096.

Araújo, Wilma Maria Coelho, Nancy de Pilla Montebelo, Raquel Braz Assunção Botelho, and Luiz Antônio Borgo. 2014. *Alquimia Dos Alimentos - Editora Senac - São Paulo*. Edited by SENAC. 3rd ed. Brasília: SENAC.

Arruda Daguer Damasceno, Luana Rincon, Raquel Braz Assunção Botelho, and Ernandes Rodrigues de Alencar. 2020. "Development of Novel Plant-Based Milk Based on Chickpea and Coconut." *LWT*, April, 109479. https://doi.org/10.1016/j.lwt.2020.109479.

Aued-Pimentel, Sabria, Edna Emy Kumagai, Mahyara Markievicz Mancio Kus, Miriam Solange Fernandes Caruso, Mário Tavares, and Odair Zenebon. 2009. "Trans Fatty Acids in Refined Polyunsaturated Vegetable Oils Commercialized in the City of São Paulo, Brazil." *Ciencia e Tecnologia de Alimentos* 29 (3): 646–51. https://doi.org/10.1590/S0101-20612009000300030.

Azadbakht, Leila, Fahimeh Haghighatdoost, Awat Feizi, and Ahmad Esmaillzadeh. 2013. "Breakfast Eating Pattern and Its Association with Dietary Quality Indices and Anthropometric Measurements in Young Women in Isfahan." *Nutrition* 29 (2): 420–25. https://doi.org/10.1016/j.nut.2012.07.008.

Baltar, Valéria Troncoso, Diana Barbosa Cunha, Roberta De Oliveira Santos, Dirce Maria Marchioni, and Rosely Sichieri. 2018. "Breakfast Patterns and Their Association with Body Mass Index in Brazilian Adults." *Cadernos de Saude Publica* 34 (6). https://doi.org/10.1590/0102-311X00111917.

Bedani, Raquel, and Elizeu Antonio Rossi. 2005. "O Consumo de Cálcio e a Osteoporose." *Semina: Ciências Biológicas e Da Saúde* 26 (1): 3. https://doi.org/10.5433/1679-0367.2005v26n1p3. [Calcium Consumption and Osteoporosis. *Semina: Biological and Health Sciences*]

Bellisle, France, Pascale Hébel, Aurée Salmon-Legagneur, and Florent Vieux. 2018. "Breakfast Consumption in French Children, Adolescents, and Adults: A Nationally Representative Cross-Sectional Survey Examined in the Context of the International Breakfast Research Initiative." *Nutrients* 10 (8). https://doi.org/10.3390/nu10081056.

Benatar, Jocelyn R., and Ralph Ah Stewart. 2014. "The Effects of Changing Dairy Intake on Trans and Saturated Fatty Acid Levels-Results from a Randomized Controlled Study." *Nutrition Journal* 13 (1): 32. https://doi.org/10.1186/1475-2891-13-32.

Bertolino, Carla Novaes, Teresa Gontijo Castro, Daniela S. Sartorelli, Sandra R.G. Ferreira, and Marly Augusto Cardoso. 2006. "Influência Do Consumo Alimentar de Ácidos Graxos Trans No Perfil de Lipídios Séricos Em Nipo-Brasileiros de Bauru, São Paulo, Brasil." *Cadernos de Saude Publica* 22 (2): 357–64. https://doi.org/10.1590/s0102-311x2006000200013. [Influence of Food Consumption of Trans Fatty Acids on the Profile of Serum Lipids in Japanese-Brazilians from Bauru, São Paulo, Brazil. *Public Health Notebooks*]

Bispo, Janaina Sarmento, and Maria José Roncada. 2006. *Perfil Alimentar Referente ao Desjejum dos Professores da Universidade De Brasilia-UnB. Dissertação Apresentada Ao Curso de Pós-Graduação Em Nutrição Humana, Do Departamento de Nutrição Da Universidade de Brasília, Para Obtenção Do Título de Mestre Em Nut. [Food Profile Regarding the Breakfast of the Professors of the University De Brasilia-*

UnB. Dissertation Presented to the Postgraduate Course in Human Nutrition, Department of Nutrition, University of Brasilia, to obtain the title of Master in Nut.]

Bolhuis, Dieuwerke P., Elisabeth H. M. Temme, Fari T. Koeman, Martijn W. J. Noort, Stefanie Kremer, and Anke M. Janssen. 2011. "A Salt Reduction of 50% in Bread Does Not Decrease Bread Consumption or Increase Sodium Intake by the Choice of Sandwich Fillings." *The Journal of Nutrition* 141 (12): 2249–55. https://doi.org/10.3945/jn.111.141366.

Bonjour, Jean Philippe, Marius Kraenzlin, Régis Levasseur, Michelle Warren, and Susan Whiting. 2013. "Dairy in Adulthood: From Foods to Nutrient Interactions on Bone and Skeletal Muscle Health." *Journal of the American College of Nutrition*. Taylor & Francis. https://doi.org/10.1080/07315724.2013.816604.

Boom, Anneke van den, Lluís Serra-Majem, Lourdes Ribas, Joy Ngo, Carmen Pérez-Rodrigo, Javier Aranceta, and Reginald Fletcher. 2006. "The Contribution of Ready-to-Eat Cereals to Daily Nutrient Intake and Breakfast Quality in a Mediterranean Setting." *Journal of the American College of Nutrition* 25 (2): 135–43. https://doi.org/10.1080/07315724.2006.10719524.

Brasil. Ministério da Saúde. 2008. *Guia Alimentar Para a População Brasileira*. https://doi.org/978-85-334-2176-9.

Brasil, Instituto Brasileiro de Geografia e Estatística - IBGE. 2011. *Pesquisa de Orçamentos Familiares 2008-2009. IBGE. Instituto Brasileiro de Geografi a e Estatística - BRASIL*. Ministério. Vol. 39. https://doi.org/ISSN 0101-4234. [*2008-2009 Household Budget Survey. IBGE. Brazilian Institute of Geography and Statistics – BRAZIL*]

Brown, Michelle M Bohan, Jillian E Milanes, David B Allison, and Andrew W Brown. 2017. "Eating Compared to Skipping Breakfast Has No Discernible Benefit for Obesity-Related Anthropometrics: Systematic Review and Meta-Analysis of Randomized Controlled Trials." *The FASEB Journal* 31 (1_supplement): lb363–lb363. https://doi.org/10.1096/fasebj.31.1_supplement.lb363.

Bueno, Aline L., and Mauro A. Czepielewski. 2008. "A Importância Do Consumo Dietético de Cálcio e Vitamina D No Crescimento." *Jornal de Pediatria*. Sociedade Brasileira de Pediatria. https://doi.org/10.2223/JPED.1816. [The Importance of Dietary Consumption of Calcium and Vitamin D in Growth. *Journal of Pediatrics*.]

Cardoso, Letícia de Oliveira, Elyne Montenegro Engstrom, Iuri da Costa Leite, and Inês Rugani Ribeiro de Castro. 2009. "Fatores Socioeconômicos, Demográficos, Ambientais e Comportamentais Associados Ao Excesso de Peso Em Adolescentes: Uma Revisão Siste-mática Da Literatura." *Revista Brasileira de Epidemiologia* 12 (3): 378–403. https://doi.org/10.1590/s1415-790x2009000300008. ["Socioeconomic, Demographic, Environmental and Behavioral Factors Associated with Overweight in Adolescents: A Systematic Review of Literature." *Brazilian Journal of Epidemiology*]

Carrijo, Alinne, Raquel Botelho, Rita Akutsu, Renata Zandonadi, Alinne de Paula Carrijo, Raquel Braz Assunção Botelho, Rita de Cássia Coelho de Almeida Akutsu, and Renata Puppin Zandonadi. 2018. "Is What Low-Income Brazilians Are Eating in Popular Restaurants Contributing to Promote Their Health?" *Nutrients* 10 (4): 414. https://doi.org/10.3390/nu10040414.

Carrillo-Larco, Rodrigo M, and Antonio Bernabe-Ortiz. 2020. "Sodium and Salt Consumption in Latin America and the Caribbean: A Systematic-Review and Meta-Analysis of Population-Based Studies and Surveys." *Nutrients* 12 (2): 556. https://doi.org/10.3390/nu12020556.

Castro, Michelle Alessandra de, Rodrigo Ribeiro Barros, Milena Baptista Bueno, Chester Luiz Galvão César, and Regina Mara Fisberg. 2009. "Trans Fatty Acid Intake among the Population of the City of São Paulo, Brazil." *Revista de Saúde Pública* 43 (6): 991–97. https://doi.org/10.1590/s0034-89102009005000084.

Cho, Sungsoo, Marion Dietrich, Coralie J.P. Brown, Celeste A. Clark, and Gladys Block. 2003. "The Effect of Breakfast Type on Total Daily Energy Intake and Body Mass Index: Results from the Third National Health and Nutrition Examination Survey (Nhanes Iii)." *Journal of the*

American College of Nutrition 22 (4): 296–302. https://doi.org/ 10.1080/07315724.2003.10719307.

Cortés, E., M. J. Aguilar Cordero, M. M. Rizo, and M. J. Hidalgo. 2013. "Ácidos Grasos Transen La Nutrición de Niños Con Trastornos Neurológicos." *Nutricion Hospitalaria* 28 (4): 1140–44. https://doi.org/10.3305/nh.2013.28.4.6527. [Trans Fatty Acids The Nutrition Of Children With Neurological Disorders. *Hospital Nutrition*]

Costa Proença, Rossana Pacheco Da, and Bruna Maria Silveira. 2012. "Recomendações de Ingestão e Rotulagem de Gordura Trans Em Alimentos Industrializados Brasileiros: Análise de Documentos Ofi Ciais." *Revista de Saude Publica* 46 (5): 923–28. https://doi.org/ 10.1590/S0034-89102012000500020. ["Recommendations for Ingestion and Labeling of Trans Fat in Brazilian Industrialized Foods: Analysis of Official Documents." *Public Health Magazine*]

Deshmukh-Taskar, Priya, Theresa A Nicklas, John D Radcliffe, Carol E O'Neil, and Yan Liu. 2013. "The Relationship of Breakfast Skipping and Type of Breakfast Consumed with Overweight/Obesity, Abdominal Obesity, Other Cardiometabolic Risk Factors and the Metabolic Syndrome in Young Adults. The National Health and Nutrition Examination Survey (NHANES):" *Public Health Nutrition* 16 (11): 2073–82. https://doi.org/10.1017/S1368980012004296.

Díaz-Torrente, Ximena, and Daiana Quintiliano-Scarpelli. 2020. "Dietary Patterns of Breakfast Consumption among Chilean University Students." *Nutrients* 12 (2). https://doi.org/10.3390/nu12020552.

Drewnowski, Adam, Colin D. Rehm, and Florent Vieux. 2018. "Breakfast in the United States: Food and Nutrient Intakes in Relation to Diet Quality in National Health and Examination Survey 2011–2014. a Study from the International Breakfast Research Initiative." *Nutrients* 10 (9). https://doi.org/10.3390/nu10091200.

Durá Travé, T. 2013. "Análisis Nutricional Del Desayuno y Almuerzo En Una Población Universitaria." *Nutrición Hospitalaria* 28 (4): 1291–99. https://doi.org/10.3305/nh.2013.28.4.6479. [Nutritional Analysis of Breakfast and Lunch in a University Population. *Hospital Nutrition*]

Enes, Carla Cristina, and Betzabeth Slater. 2010. "Obesidade Na Adolescência e Seus Principais Fatores Determinantes." *Revista Brasileira de Epidemiologia*. Associação Brasileira de Saúde Coletiva. https://doi.org/10.1590/s1415-790x2010000100015. [Adolescent Obesity and Its Main Determining Factors. *Brazilian Journal of Epidemiology*.]

Fagt, Sisse, Jeppe Matthiessen, Camilla Thyregod, Karsten Kørup, and Anja Biltoft-Jensen. 2018. "Breakfast in Denmark. Prevalence of Consumption, Intake of Foods, Nutrients and Dietary Quality. a Study from the International Breakfast Research Initiative." *Nutrients* 10 (8). https://doi.org/10.3390/nu10081085.

Fayet-Moore, Flavia, Andrew McConnell, Kate Tuck, and Peter Petocz. 2017. "Breakfast and Breakfast Cereal Choice and Its Impact on Nutrient and Sugar Intakes and Anthropometric Measures among a Nationally Representative Sample of Australian Children and Adolescents." *Nutrients* 9 (10). https://doi.org/10.3390/nu9101045.

Fernández Morales, I., M. V. Aguilar Vilas, C. J. Mateos Vega, and M. C. Martínez Para. 2011. "Breakfast Quality and Its Relationship to the Prevalence of Overweight and Obesity in Adolescents in Guadalajara (Spain)." *Nutricion Hospitalaria* 26 (5): 952–58. https://doi.org/10.1590/S0212-16112011000500005.

Freitas, Patrícia Pinheiro de, Raquel de Deus Mendonça, and Aline Cristine Souza Lopes. 2013. "Factors Associated with Breakfasting in Users of a Public Health Service." *Revista de Nutrição* 26 (2): 195–203. https://doi.org/10.1590/S1415-52732013000200007.

Galas, Aleksander, Malgorzata Augustyniak, and Elzbieta Sochacka-Tatara. 2013. "Does Dietary Calcium Interact with Dietary Fiber against Colorectal Cancer? A Case-Control Study in Central Europe." *Nutrition Journal* 12 (October): 134. https://doi.org/10.1186/1475-2891-12-134.

Gibney, Michael J., Susan I. Barr, France Bellisle, Adam Drewnowski, Sisse Fagt, Sinead Hopkins, Barbara Livingstone, et al. 2018. "Towards an Evidence-Based Recommendation for a Balanced Breakfast—A Proposal from the International Breakfast Research Initiative." *Nutrients* 10 (10). https://doi.org/10.3390/nu10101540.

Gibney, Michael J., Susan I. Barr, France Bellisle, Adam Drewnowski, Sisse Fagt, Barbara Livingstone, Gabriel Masset, et al. 2018. "Breakfast in Human Nutrition: The International Breakfast Research Initiative." *Nutrients*. MDPI AG. https://doi.org/10.3390/nu10050559.

Gibson, Sigrid, and Margaret Ashwell. 2011. "Dietary Patterns among British Adults: Compatibility with Dietary Guidelines for Salt/Sodium, Fat, Saturated Fat and Sugars." *Public Health Nutrition* 14 (8): 1323–36. https://doi.org/10.1017/S1368980011000875.

Ginani, Verônica Cortez Veronica Cortez V.C C, J.S S Janini Selva Ginani, R.B.A Raquel Braz Assunçúo Assunção Assuncao R.B.A Raquel Braz Assunçúo Assunção Assuncao Botelho, Renata Puppin Zandonadi, Rita C.C. C A de Cássia Cassia Cássia Akutsu, Wilma Maria Coelho Araújo, Rita De Cássia Akutsu, et al. 2010. "Reducing Fat Content of Brazilian Traditional Preparations Does Not Alter Food Acceptance: Development of a Model for Fat Reduction That Conciliates Health and Culture." *Journal of Culinary Science & Technology* 8 (4): 229–41. https://doi.org/10.1080/15428052.
2011.535758.

Giuseppe, R. di, A. Di Castelnuovo, C. Melegari, F. De Lucia, I. Santimone, A. Sciarretta, P. Barisciano, et al. 2012. "Typical Breakfast Food Consumption and Risk Factors for Cardiovascular Disease in a Large Sample of Italian Adults." *Nutrition, Metabolism and Cardiovascular Diseases* 22 (4): 347–54. https://doi.org/10.1016/j.numecd.
2010.07.006.

Hallström, Lena, Idoia Labayen, Jonatan R. Ruiz, Emma Patterson, Carine A. Vereecken, Christina Breidenassel, Frédéric Gottrand, et al. 2013. "Breakfast Consumption and CVD Risk Factors in European Adolescents: The HELENA (Healthy Lifestyle in Europe by Nutrition in Adolescence) Study." *Public Health Nutrition* 16 (7): 1296–1305. https://doi.org/10.1017/S1368980012000973.

Hallström, Lena, Carine A. Vereecken, Jonatan R. Ruiz, Emma Patterson, Chantal C. Gilbert, Giovina Catasta, Ligia Esperanza Díaz, et al. 2011. "Breakfast Habits and Factors Influencing Food Choices at Breakfast in Relation to Socio-Demographic and Family Factors among European

Adolescents. The HELENA Study." *Appetite* 56 (3): 649–57. https://doi.org/10.1016/j.appet.2011.02.019.

Harter, Daniele Lazzarotto, Fernanda Michielin Busnello, Raquel Papandreus I. Dibi, Airton Tetelbom Stein, Sérgio Kakuta Kato, and Carla Maria De Martini Vanin. 2013. "Associação Entre Baixa Massa Óssea e Ingestão de Cálcio e Cafeína Em Mulheres Climatéricas Na Região Sul Do Brasil: Estudo Transversal." *Sao Paulo Medical Journal* 131 (5): 315–22. https://doi.org/10.1590/1516-3180.2013.1315428. [Association Between Low Bone Mass and Calcium and Caffeine Intake in Climacteric Women in Southern Brazil: Cross-Sectional Study. *Sao Paulo Medical Journal*]

Hassan, Bruna Kulik, Diana Barbosa Cunha, Gloria Valeria da Veiga, Rosangela Alves Pereira, and Rosely Sichieri. 2018. "Changes in Breakfast Frequency and Composition during Adolescence: The Adolescent Nutritional Assessment Longitudinal Study, a Cohort from Brazil." *PLoS ONE* 13 (7). https://doi.org/10.1371/journal.pone.0200587.

Herrera, J. R. 2007. "Caracterización Del Consumo Deficitario de Los Grupos Básicos de Alimentos En El Estudiante de Cuarto Año En La Escuela de Medicina "Dr. Witremundo Torrealba". Maracay, Venezuela." *Comunidad y Salud* 5 (2). [Characterization of Deficient Consumption of Basic Food Groups in Fourth Year Student at the School of Medicine Dr. Witremundo Torrealba. Maracay, Venezuela. *Community and Health*]

Higdon, Jane V., and Balz Frei. 2006. "Coffee and Health: A Review of Recent Human Research." *Critical Reviews in Food Science and Nutrition* 46 (2): 101–23. https://doi.org/10.1080/10408390500400009.

Höfelmann, Doroteia Aparecida, and Nayara Momm. 2014. "Café Da Manhã: Omissão e Fatores Associados Em Escolares de Itajaí, Santa Catarina, Brasil." *Nutrire* 39 (1): 40–55. https://doi.org/10.4322/nutrire.2014.005. ["Breakfast: Omission and Associated Factors in Schoolchildren from Itajaí, Santa Catarina, Brazil."]

Hoyland, Alexa, Louise Dye, and Clare L. Lawton. 2009. "A Systematic Review of the Effect of Breakfast on the Cognitive Performance of

Children and Adolescents." *Nutrition Research Reviews.* https://doi.org/10.1017/S0954422409990175.

Huang, Ru Yi, Chuan Chin Huang, Frank B. Hu, and Jorge E. Chavarro. 2016. "Vegetarian Diets and Weight Reduction: A Meta-Analysis of Randomized Controlled Trials." *Journal of General Internal Medicine* 31 (1): 109–16. https://doi.org/10.1007/s11606-015-3390-7.

Idec. 2015. *Redução de Sódio Em Alimentos: Uma Análise Dos Acordos Voluntários No Brasil | Idec - Instituto Brasileiro de Defesa Do Consumidor.* [Reduction of Sodium in Food: An Analysis of Voluntary Agreements in Brazil | Idec - Brazilian Institute for Consumer Protection.]

Ignácio, Ana Karoline Ferreira, José Tarcísio de Domenico Rodrigues, Patrícia Yuasa Niizu, Yoon Kil Chang, and Caroline Joy Stell. 2013. "Efeito Da Substituição de Cloreto de Sódio Por Cloreto de Potássio Em Pão Francês." *Brazilian Journal of Food Technology* 16 (1): 01–11. https://doi.org/10.1590/s1981-67232013005000010.

Iqbal, K., L. Schwingshackl, M. Gottschald, S. Knüppel, M. Stelmach-Mardas, K. Aleksandrova, and H. Boeing. 2017. "Breakfast Quality and Cardiometabolic Risk Profiles in an Upper Middle-Aged German Population." *European Journal of Clinical Nutrition* 71 (11): 1312–20. https://doi.org/10.1038/ejcn.2017.116.

Jomori, Manuela Mika, Rossana Pacheco da Costa Proença, and Maria Cristina Marino Calvo. 2008. "Determinantes de Escolha Alimentar." *Revista de Nutrição* 21 (1): 63–73. https://doi.org/10.1590/S1415-52732008000100007. [Determinants of Food Choice. *Nutrition Magazine*]

Kubota, Yasuhiko, Hiroyasu Iso, Norie Sawada, and Shoichiro Tsugane. 2016. "Association of Breakfast Intake with Incident Stroke and Coronary Heart Disease: The Japan Public Health Center-Based Study." *Stroke* 47 (2): 477–81. https://doi.org/10.1161/STROKEAHA.115.011350.

Laissa, Ana, O Aguiar, Clarissa Marques Maranhão, Lívia Carvalho Spinelli, Roberta Marinho De Figueiredo, Jussara Melo, C Maia, Rosane Costa Gomes, Hélcio De, and Sousa Maranhão. 2013. "Artigo Original

Avaliação Clínica e Evolutiva de Crianças Em Programa de Atendimento Ao Uso de Fórmulas Para Alergia à Proteína Do Leite de Vaca Clinical and Follow up Assessment of Children in a Program Directed at the Use of Formulas for Cow's Milk Prot." *Rev Paul Pediatr*. Vol. 31. ["Original Article Clinical and Evolutionary Evaluation of Children in a Program to Assist the Use of Formulas for Cow's Milk Protein Allergy Clinical and Follow up Assessment of Children in a Program Directed at the Use of Formulas for Cow's Milk Prot." *Rev Paul Pediatr.*]

Leal, Greisse Viero da Silva, Sonia Tucunduva Philippi, Sandra Marcela Mahecha Matsudo, and Erika Christiane Toassa. 2010. "Consumo Alimentar e Padrão de Refeições de Adolescentes, São Paulo, Brasil." *Revista Brasileira de Epidemiologia* 13 (3): 457–67. https://doi.org/10.1590/s1415-790x2010000300009. ["Food Consumption and Meal Pattern of Adolescents, São Paulo, Brazil." *Brazilian Journal of Epidemiology*]

Luz, Andréa Ribeiro. 2007. *Concentrações Séricas de Cálcio e Ferro Em Jovens Consumidores de Tereré (Ilex Paraguariensis), Dourados-MS*. University of Brasília. [*Serum concentrations of calcium and iron in young consumers of Tereré (Ilex Paraguariensis), Dourados-MS.*]

Maeda, Sergio Setsuo, Victoria Z.C. Borba, Marília Brasilio Rodrigues Camargo, Dalisbor Marcelo Weber Silva, João Lindolfo Cunha Borges, Francisco Bandeira, and Marise Lazaretti-Castro. 2014. "Recommendations of the Brazilian Society of Endocrynology and Metabolism for the Diagnose and Treatment of Vitamin D Deficiency. (Recomendações Da Sociedade Brasileira de Endocrinologia e Metabologia (SBEM) Para o Diagnóstico e Tratamento Da Hipovitaminose D.") *Arquivos Brasileiros de Endocrinologia e Metabologia* 58 (5): 411–33. https://doi.org/10.1590/0004-2730000003388.

Marangoni, Franca, Andrea Poli, Carlo Agostoni, Pasquale Di Pietro, Claudio Cricelli, Ovidio Brignoli, Giuseppe Fatati, et al. 2009. "A Consensus Document on the Role of Breakfast in the Attainment and

Maintenance of Health and Wellness." *Acta Bio-Medica: Atenei Parmensis* 80 (2): 166–71.

Melby, Melissa K., and Wakako Takeda. 2014. "Lifestyle Constraints, Not Inadequate Nutrition Education, Cause Gap between Breakfast Ideals and Realities among Japanese in Tokyo." *Appetite* 72 (January): 37–49. https://doi.org/10.1016/j.appet.2013.09.013.

Melo, Martha Teresa Siqueira Marques, Ana Claudia Carvalho Moura, Maria das Dôres Cavalcante dos Santos, Bianca Lourrany dos Santos Silva, Ivone Freires de Oliveira Costa Nunes, Suely Carvalho Santiago Barreto, Marize Melo dos Santos, Suzana Maria Rebêlo Sampaio da Paz, and Cecilia Maria Resende Gonçalves de Carvalho. 2020. "Public Market Breakfast: A Food Tradition." *Journal of Food and Nutrition Research, Vol. 8, 2020, Pages 74-79* 8 (2): 74–79. https://doi.org/10.12691/JFNR-8-2-1.

Meneton, P., L. Lafay, A. Tard, A. Dufour, J. Ireland, J. Ménard, and J. L. Volatier. 2009. "Dietary Sources and Correlates of Sodium and Potassium Intakes in the French General Population." *European Journal of Clinical Nutrition* 63 (10): 1169–75. https://doi.org/10.1038/ejcn.2009.57.

Min, Chanyang, Hwayoung Noh, Yun Sook Kang, Hea Jin Sim, Hyun Wook Baik, Won O. Song, Jihyun Yoon, Young Hee Park, and Hyojee Joung. 2012. "Breakfast Patterns Are Associated with Metabolic Syndrome in Korean Adults." *Nutrition Research and Practice* 6 (1): 61–67. https://doi.org/10.4162/nrp.2012.6.1.61.

Monteagudo, Celia, Alba Palacín-Arce, Maria Del Mar Bibiloni, Antoni Pons, Josep A. Tur, Fatima Olea-Serrano, and Miguel Mariscal-Arcas. 2013. "Proposal for a Breakfast Quality Index (BQI) for Children and Adolescents." *Public Health Nutrition* 16 (4): 639–44. https://doi.org/10.1017/S1368980012003175.

Monteiro, Luana Silva, Amanda de Moura Souza, Bruna Kulik Hassan, Camilla Chermont Prochnik Estima, Rosely Sichieri, and Rosangela Alves Pereira. 2017a. "Breakfast Eating among Brazilian Adolescents: Analysis of the National Dietary Survey 2008-2009." *Revista de*

Nutricao 30 (4): 463–76. https://doi.org/10.1590/1678-98652017 00400006.

———. 2017b. "Breakfast Eating among Brazilian Adolescents: Analysis of the National Dietary Survey 2008-2009." *Revista de Nutrição* 30 (4): 463–76. https://doi.org/10.1590/1678-98652017000400006.

Morais, Glaucia Queiroz, and Maria Goretti Pessoa de Araújo Burgos. 2007. "Impacto Dos Nutrientes Na Saúde Óssea: Novas Tendências." *Revista Brasileira de Ortopedia* 42 (7): 189–94. https://doi.org/10.1590/s0102-36162007000700002. [Impact of Nutrients on Bone Health: New Trends. *Brazilian Journal of Orthopedics*]

Moura Souza, Amanda de, Ilana Nogueira Bezerra, Rosangela Alves Pereira, Karen Eileen Peterson, and Rosely Sichieri. 2013. "Dietary Sources of Sodium Intake in Brazil in 2008-2009." *Journal of the Academy of Nutrition and Dietetics* 113 (10): 1359–65.

Mozaffarian, Dariush, Saman Fahimi, Gitanjali M. Singh, Renata Micha, Shahab Khatibzadeh, Rebecca E. Engell, Stephen Lim, Goodarz Danaei, Majid Ezzati, and John Powles. 2014. "Global Sodium Consumption and Death from Cardiovascular Causes." *New England Journal of Medicine* 371 (7): 624–34. https://doi.org/10.1056/NEJMoa1304127.

Nestel, Paul. 2014. "Trans Fatty Acids: Are Its Cardiovascular Risks Fully Appreciated?" *Clinical Therapeutics*. Excerpta Medica Inc. https://doi.org/10.1016/j.clinthera.2014.01.020.

Nicklas, Theresa A., Leann Myers, Christina Reger, Bettina Beech, and Gerald S. Berenson. 1998. "Impact of Breakfast Consumption on Nutritional Adequacy of the Diets of Young Adults in Bogalusa, Louisiana: Ethnic and Gender Contrasts." *Journal of the American Dietetic Association* 98 (12): 1432–38. https://doi.org/10.1016/S0002-8223(98)00325-3.

Nurul-Fadhilah, Abdullah, Pey Sze Teo, Inge Huybrechts, and Leng Huat Foo. 2013. "Infrequent Breakfast Consumption Is Associated with Higher Body Adiposity and Abdominal Obesity in Malaysian School-Aged Adolescents." Edited by Olga Y. Gorlova. *PLoS ONE* 8 (3): e59297. https://doi.org/10.1371/journal.pone.0059297.

O'Neil, Carol E., Carol Byrd-Bredbenner, Dayle Hayes, Laura Jana, Sylvia E. Klinger, and Susan Stephenson-Martin. 2014. "The Role of Breakfast in Health: Definition and Criteria for a Quality Breakfast." *Journal of the Academy of Nutrition and Dietetics* 114 (12): S8–26. https://doi.org/10.1016/j.jand.2014.08.022.

Pedersen, Trine P., Charlotte Meilstrup, Bjørn E. Holstein, and Mette Rasmussen. 2012. "Fruit and Vegetable Intake Is Associated with Frequency of Breakfast, Lunch and Evening Meal: Cross-Sectional Study of 11-, 13-, and 15-Year-Olds." *International Journal of Behavioral Nutrition and Physical Activity* 9 (February): 9. https://doi.org/10.1186/1479-5868-9-9.

Pereira, Giselle A.P., Patricia S. Genaro, Marcelo M. Pinheiro, Vera L. Szejnfeld, and Ligia A. Martini. 2009. "Dietary Calcium - Strategies to Optimize Intake." *Revista Brasileira de Reumatologia*. https://doi.org/10.1590/S0482-50042009000200008.

Pereira, Mark A., Elizabeth Erickson, Patricia McKee, Karilyn Schrankler, Susan K. Raatz, Leslie A. Lytle, and Anthony D. Pellegrini. 2011. "Breakfast Frequency and Quality May Affect Glycemia and Appetite in Adults and Children." *The Journal of Nutrition* 141 (1): 163–68. https://doi.org/10.3945/jn.109.114405.

Pineli, Lívia L O de L. de O., Raquel B.A. A Botelho, Renata P. Zandonadi, Juliana L. Solorzano, Guilherme T. de Oliveira, Caio Eduardo G. Reis, and Danielle da S. Teixeira. 2015. "Low Glycemic Index and Increased Protein Content in a Novel Quinoa Milk." *LWT - Food Science and Technology* 63 (2): 1261–67. https://doi.org/10.1016/j.lwt.2015.03.094.

Proença, R. P. C. 2010. Food and Globalization: Some Reflections ("Alimentação e Globalização: Algumas Reflexões."). *Ciência e Cultura (Science and Culture)* 62 (4): 43–47.

Proença, Rossana Pacheco da Costa, Anete Araújo Sousa, Marcela Boro Veiros, and Bethania Hering. 2005. *Qualidade Nutricional e Sensorial Na Produção de Refeições*. Florianópolis: UFSC. [*Nutritional and Sensory Quality in Meal Production.*]

Ruiz, Emma, José Manuel Ávila, Teresa Valero, Paula Rodriguez, and Gregorio Varela-Moreiras. 2018. "*Breakfast Consumption in Spain:*

Patterns, Nutrient Intake and Quality. Findings from the ANIBES Study, a Study from the International Breakfast Research Initiative." *Nutrients* 10 (9). https://doi.org/10.3390/nu10091324.

Sarno, Flavio, Rafael Moreira Claro, Renata Bertazzi Levy, Daniel Henrique Bandoni, Sandra Roberta Gouvêa Ferreira, and Carlos Augusto Monteiro. 2009. "[Estimated Sodium Intake by the Brazilian Population, 2002-2003]." *Revista de Saude Publica* 43 (2): 219–25.

Scheen, André J, and Luc F Van Gaal. 2014. "Combating the Dual Burden: Therapeutic Targeting of Common Pathways in Obesity and Type 2 Diabetes." *The Lancet Diabetes & Endocrinology* 2 (11): 911–22. https://doi.org/10.1016/S2213-8587(14)70004-X.

Schusdziarra, Volker, Margit Hausmann, Claudia Wittke, Johanna Mittermeier, Marietta Kellner, Aline Naumann, Stefan Wagenpfeil, and Johannes Erdmann. 2011. "Impact of Breakfast on Daily Energy Intake - An Analysis of Absolute versus Relative Breakfast Calories." *Nutrition Journal* 10 (1): 5. https://doi.org/10.1186/1475-2891-10-5.

Sethi, Swati, S. K. Tyagi, and Rahul K. Anurag. 2016. "Plant-Based Milk Alternatives an Emerging Segment of Functional Beverages: A Review." *Journal of Food Science and Technology*. Springer India. https://doi.org/10.1007/s13197-016-2328-3.

Sievert, Katherine, Sultana Monira Hussain, Matthew J. Page, Yuanyuan Wang, Harrison J. Hughes, Mary Malek, and Flavia M. Cicuttini. 2019. "Effect of Breakfast on Weight and Energy Intake: Systematic Review and Meta-Analysis of Randomised Controlled Trials." *BMJ (Online)* 364 (January). https://doi.org/10.1136/bmj.l42.

Soares, M. J., and W. Chan She Ping-Delfos. 2008. "Second Meal Effects of Dietary Calcium and Vitamin D." *European Journal of Clinical Nutrition* 62 (7): 872–78. https://doi.org/10.1038/sj.ejcn.1602803.

Sousa, Janice Ramos de, Raquel B. A. Botelho, Rita de Cássia C. A. Akutsu, and Renata Puppin Zandonadi. 2019. "Nutritional Quality of Breakfast Consumed by the Low-Income Population in Brazil: A Nationwide Cross-Sectional Survey." *Nutrients* 11 (6): 1418. https://doi.org/10.3390/nu11061418.

Souza, A. M., R. A. Pereira, E. M. Yokoo, R. B. Levy, and R. Sichieri. 2013. "Most Consumed Foods in Brazil: National Dietary Survey 2008-2009." *Rev Saúde Pública* 47 (1): 190S-9S.

Souza, F. M., C. N. Ferrari, C. Pascotini, and F. Navarro. 2007. "Relação Entre o Índice de Massa Corporal e o Tipo de Desjejum de Pacientes de Um Consultório de Nutrição | RBONE - Revista Brasileira de Obesidade, Nutrição e Emagrecimento." *Revista Brasileira de Obesidade, Nutriçãoe Emagrecimento* 1 (3).

Spence, Charles. 2017. "Breakfast: The Most Important Meal of the Day?" *International Journal of Gastronomy and Food Science* 8 (January): 1–6. https://doi.org/10.1016/j.ijgfs.2017.01.003.

Strazzullo, P., G. Cairella, A. Campanozzi, M. Carcea, D. Galeone, F. Galletti, S. Giampaoli, L. Iacoviello, and L. Scalfi. 2012. "Population Based Strategy for Dietary Salt Intake Reduction: Italian Initiatives in the European Framework." *Nutrition, Metabolism and Cardiovascular Diseases*. https://doi.org/10.1016/j.numecd.2011.10.004.

Szajewska, Hania, and Marek Ruszczyński. 2010. "Systematic Review Demonstrating That Breakfast Consumption Influences Body Weight Outcomes in Children and Adolescents in Europe." *Critical Reviews in Food Science and Nutrition* 50 (2): 113–19. https://doi.org/10.1080/10408390903467514.

Trancoso, Suelen Caroline, Suzi Barletto Cavalli, and Rossana Pacheco da Costa Proença. 2010. "Café Da Manhã: Caracterização, Consumo e Importância Para a Saúde." *Revista de Nutrição* 23 (5): 859–69. https://doi.org/10.1590/S1415-52732010000500016. ["Breakfast: Characterization, Consumption and Importance for Health." *Nutrition Magazine*]

Triches, Rozane Márcia, and Elsa Regina Justo Giugliani. 2005. "Obesidade, Práticas Alimentares e Conhecimentos de Nutrição Em Escolares." *Revista de Saude Publica* 39 (4): 541–47. https://doi.org/10.1590/s0034-89102005000400004. ["Obesity, Eating Practices and Nutrition Knowledge in Schoolchildren." *Public Health Magazine*]

Vieira, M. V., I. R. L. Del Ciampo, and L. A. Del Ciampo. 2014. "Hábitos e Consumo Alimentar Entre Adolescentes Eutróficos e Com Excesso de

Peso." *Rev. Bras. Crescimento Desenvolv. Hum* 24 (2). ["Habits and Food Consumption Among Eutrophic and Overweight Adolescents." *Rev. Bras. Development Growth Hmm*]

Wang, Yao Fen, Su Ping Chen, Yi Ching Lee, and Chen Tsang (Simon) Tsai. 2013. "Developing Green Management Standards for Restaurants: An Application of Green Supply Chain Management." *International Journal of Hospitality Management* 34 (1): 263–73. https://doi.org/10.1016/j.ijhm.2013.04.001.

Williams, Peter G. 2014. "The Benefits of Breakfast Cereal Consumption: A Systematic Review of the Evidence Base." *Advances in Nutrition* 5 (5): 636S-673S. https://doi.org/10.3945/an.114.006247.

World Health Organization (WHO). 2011. *"Review and Updating of Current WHO Recommendations on Salt/Sodium and Potassium Consumption Call for Public Comments."*

Yoo, Ki Bong, Hee Jae Suh, Minjee Lee, Jae Hyun Kim, Jeoung A. Kwon, and Eun Cheol Park. 2014. "Breakfast Eating Patterns and the Metabolic Syndrome: The Korea National Health and Nutrition Examination Survey (KNHANES) 2007-2009." *Asia Pacific Journal of Clinical Nutrition* 23 (1): 128–37. https://doi.org/10.6133/apjcn.2014.23.1.08.

Zakrzewski-Fruer, Julia K., Tatiana Plekhanova, Dafni Mandila, Yannis Lekatis, and Keith Tolfrey. 2017. "Effect of Breakfast Omission and Consumption on Energy Intake and Physical Activity in Adolescent Girls: A Randomised Controlled Trial." *British Journal of Nutrition* 118 (5): 392–400. https://doi.org/10.1017/S0007114517002148.

Zandonadi, Renata Puppin, Raquel B A Botelho, Verônica C Ginani, Rita De Cássia, C A Akutsu, Karin Eleonora De Oliveira Savio, and Wilma M C Araújo. 2014. *Sodium and Health: New Proposal of Distribution for Major Meals* 6 (3): 195–201. https://doi.org/10.4236/health.2014.63029.

In: Breakfast
Editor: Petr Měchura

ISBN: 978-1-53618-500-3
© 2020 Nova Science Publishers, Inc.

Chapter 2

POTENTIAL BENEFITS OF CHOOSING PLANT-BASED MEALS FOR BREAKFAST

Shila Minari Hargreaves[*],
Raquel Braz Assunção Botelho
and Renata Puppin Zandonadi
Department of Nutrition, University of Brasília, Brasília, DF, Brazil

ABSTRACT

Evidence shows that eating breakfast has positive effects on health, mainly due to better food intake during the day and hormonal profile. However, the nutritional quality of the meal must be taken into account to guarantee these health benefits. Over the last years, health professionals, studies, and media have put effort into encouraging a reduction of refined carbohydrates intake (sugary cereals, white bread, and sugary beverages such as artificial juices or milk chocolate), considering a traditional western diet breakfast. Despite a potential positive effect of reducing sugar and refined foods intake in health, breakfast recommendations have shifted towards more animal-based meals, which include eggs, bacon, cheese, and even coffee with butter (bulletproof coffee). In the short-term, these foods might indeed bring some benefits, such as lower ghrelin levels (resulting in more satiety) and lower post-prandial glycemic peaks. On the other hand, a single high saturated fat meal or high animal protein meal can increase inflammatory markers over the following hours and the risk of non-communicable diseases and mortality, leading to worse gut microbiome profile. A fiber plant-based meal can have better effects on health, equally contributing to satiety and, at the same time, helping to reduce inflammatory markers and improve microbiome health. A breakfast based on fruits, vegetables, and whole grains, such as oatmeal or whole-grain bread, can lead to a more favorable lipid profile, contributing to diabetes and overweight prevention and control, without the harmful effects of eating sugary industrialized foods. It is essential to stimulate the consumption of breakfast and a higher intake of calories during the morning period compared to night time. However, the use of whole-foods plant-based breakfast should be encouraged instead of an animal-based meal to guarantee long-term health benefits.

Keywords: plant-based, breakfast, vegetarian, vegan

INTRODUCTION

It has already been described that the habit of eating breakfast is associated with better health outcomes. Breakfast skipping, as well as eating more calories during later day time, results in worse hormonal profile (including ghrelin, insulin, and melatonin), glucose and lipid levels, and increases the risk of type 2 diabetes and heart disease (Henry, Kaur, and Quek 2020; Uzhova et al. 2017).

More studies in the field of Chrono-nutrition have been emerging over the last years, showing the relevance of meal timing on our metabolism and health. Higher caloric intake during breakfast results in more significant weight loss and lower daily glucose, insulin, ghrelin, and hunger scores than a higher caloric intake during dinner in isocaloric diets. Besides weight gain, late eating leads to circadian rhythms dysfunction, deregulating appetite, and sleep hormones, as well as metabolic dysfunction (Kessler and Pivovarova-Ramich 2019). Moreover, since skipping breakfast can increase hunger throughout the day, individuals who do not eat breakfast might compensate it by eating more calories later, increasing the chances of snacking and binging. More unhealthy food choices have been observed among individuals who skip breakfast, and this habit was also associated with a higher prevalence of atherosclerosis (Uzhova et al. 2017).

A meta-analysis of observational studies found a 22% and 15% increased risk of type 2 diabetes on breakfast-skippers on cohort and cross-sectional studies, respectively. The higher satiating effect and lower appetite experienced by those who eat breakfast could be critical protective factors (Bi et al. 2015). Moreover, a more detailed analysis revealed a dose-response effect. Each day per week of skipping breakfast increases the risk of type 2 diabetes, reaching a peak of 55% higher risk with 4-5 days. This result was partially influenced by the body mass index (BMI) since the increased risk dropped to 40% after adjustment (Ballon, Neuenschwander, and Schlesinger 2018).

Despite the described positive health effects related to breakfast intake, it is also relevant to take into account the meal quality to establish targeted recommendations to the population to include breakfast daily. If individuals who do not regularly eat breakfast are stimulated to eat in the morning but base this meal on knowingly unhealthy foods, the potential health benefits might be impaired, and this new habit could even lead to worse health outcomes. Therefore, establishing the ideal foods that should compose the breakfast meal is essential to obtain the desired health and wellbeing benefits. In this sense, there are several dietary patterns influencing breakfast, in which vegetarianism has been growing and standing out (Inteligência 2018; Touvier et al. 2017).

Vegetarian dietary patterns vary according to the food restriction degree, influenced by cultural, religious, regional, and individual factors (Academy of Nutrition and Dietetics 2016; D. E. Slywitch 2015). Therefore, vegetarians are classified as those who exclude from their diet meat, poultry, fish, and their byproducts, with or without dairy products and eggs' consumption (E. Slywitch 2012). Especially over the last years, vegetarianism has gained more visibility and followers. Worldwide, Asia is the continent with the highest prevalence (19%) followed by Africa and the Middle East's (16%), South and Central America (8%), North America (6%), and Europe (5%) (Statista 2016).

A vegetarian diet can be classified according to the exclusion or not of food or food groups. A semi-vegetarian or a flexitarian limits the consumption of meat to once a week or does not consume red meat. In contrast, the pescatarian excludes all meats except fish and seafood. The lacto-ovo-vegetarian excludes all types of meats, but not eggs and dairy products. The type of vegetarian diet that excludes all foods from animal origin is the restricted vegetarian or vegan (Clarys et al. 2014; McEvoy and Woodside 2015).

Despite the progress related to the knowledge about vegetarianism, and the fast growth of its adoption, food selection for consumption must be adequate to compose a nutritional and pleasant meal to promote health.

VEGETARIANISM AND CHRONIC DISEASES

Chronic low-grade inflammation contributes to the onset and progression of non-communicable diseases, with dietary habits being considered important behavioral factors able to regulate inflammation. Meat-based or Western dietary patterns are associated with increased inflammation markers, while vegetable- and fruit-based patterns are linked to reduced inflammation (Barbaresko et al. 2013). Moreover, a vegetarian diet is associated with better blood lipid profiles and lower risk of chronic diseases, such as cancer, diabetes, and ischemic heart disease (Oussalah et al. 2020). A balanced vegetarian diet is characterized by a high intake of fruits, vegetables, whole grains, legumes, nuts, and seeds. All of which are considered nutrient-dense foods and are low in saturated fat and rich in fiber and phytochemicals, components that contribute to better health outcomes (Academy of Nutrition and Dietetics 2016).

The literature also described that vegetarians have better weight control, as well as lower body fat percentage when compared to omnivores. The more restricted the type of vegetarian diet, the lower the BMI (Spencer et al. 2003; Orlich and Fraser 2014; Kim, Cho, and Park 2012). It is well known that a higher BMI is a risk factor to many chronic diseases, such as diabetes, many types of cancer, chronic kidney disease, and cardiovascular disease

(Afshin et al. 2017). Therefore, better body weight control can have a protective effect against chronic diseases, and vegetarian diets can contribute to better health parameters (Oussalah et al. 2020).

A vegetarian diet is also useful in reducing cardiovascular risk. People who adopt a vegetarian diet have lower levels of systolic and diastolic blood pressure (Yokoyama et al. 2014), an essential protective factor related to cardiovascular disease. Moreover, vegetarians (especially vegans) when compared to omnivores have lower platelet aggregation and LDL-c levels (Hana Kahleova, Levin, and Barnard 2018), lower apolipoprotein B, and no differences in apolipoprotein A1 (Bradbury et al. 2014). The adoption of a raw vegan diet for four weeks has already been effectively used to reduce small-dense LDL-c and lipoprotein(a), other important parameters associated with better cardiovascular health (Najjar, Moore, and Montgomery 2018).

A vegetarian diet is also typically lower in advanced glycation end products (AGEs), which are components present in foods that promote oxidative stress and low-grade inflammation, contributing to an increased risk of cardiovascular diseases and diabetes (Chen et al. 2010). Finally, the high intake of animal products is associated with worse microbiome health and higher production of trimethylamine (TMA), a product that, when absorbed, is converted to trimethylamine oxide (TMAO) by the liver. It is considered an important contributor to the onset and progression of cardiovascular diseases (Koeth et al. 2013).

Consistent data from observational studies and clinical trials have already shown that vegetarians have a lower risk of developing type 2 diabetes (H. Kahleova and Pelikanova 2015; Hana Kahleova et al. 2018; Satija et al. 2016; Chiu et al. 2018; H. Kahleova et al. 2011). Also, the adoption of a vegetarian diet can be considered an efficient strategy for diabetes treatment. It shows better improvements in insulin sensitivity, weight control, glucose, and glycated hemoglobin levels and blood lipid levels when compared to conventional hypocaloric diets for the treatment of type 2 diabetes (H. Kahleova and Pelikanova 2015). On the other hand, consumption of animal protein has been linked to a higher risk of insulin resistance and diabetes when compared to an intake of plant protein

(Azemati et al. 2017) and a proportionally higher intake of carbohydrates or fats (Sluijs et al. 2010).

A potential contributor to this scenario is the higher intake of heme iron, which has already been correlated to higher diabetes risk (Zhao et al. 2012). Heme iron is absent in plants, coming exclusively from animal foods. Therefore, a higher heme iron intake is associated with higher animal products' consumption. Another vital contributor to a higher risk of diabetes is the fact that animal foods lack in fiber and phytochemicals, which are plant components known to contribute to a reduced risk of diabetes and other chronic diseases and to promote better control of diabetes in diagnosed patients (H. Kahleova and Pelikanova 2015). Plant proteins do not have the same harmful effect as animal proteins since plant protein sources, such as cereals, legumes, nuts, and seeds, are also good sources of fiber and phytochemicals.

Besides animal protein, consumption of saturated fat is also related to a higher risk of type 2 diabetes, since it increases inflammation and impairs insulin sensitivity (Shi et al. 2006). Therefore, meals rich in saturated fat, which comes mainly from animal food sources, might contribute to the development and poor control of diabetes. Finally, as previously described, a vegetarian diet leads to better weight control, lower body fat percentage, and it is considered a good weight loss strategy (Moore, McGrievy, and Turner-McGrievy 2015; Kim, Cho, and Park 2012).

BREAKFAST COMPOSITION

Breakfast is composed of a wide variety of foods all around the world. Cereals are considered essential components of this meal, consumed either in the form of breakfast cereals (commonly eaten with cold milk) or porridges, the last ones being considered a universal dish, made with different kinds of flours, eaten either sweet (usually with milk, honey, fruits, and spices) or savory (cooked in beef broth). Bread, another cereal-based food, is also widely spread among different cultures as an important breakfast item. Traditional breakfast foods like French toast, croissants,

English muffins, bagels, and rolls, as well as toasts with butter and jam, are present in many Western countries. Sandwiches made with cheese, and cured meats are more traditional in the United States, but also present in Scandinavian meals. Mediterranean countries usually include cheeses, fruits, and vegetables to its bread, while yeast spread is typical in Australia and New Zealand. Other variations of flour-based foods consumed in Western countries include pancakes and waffles, with recipes varying across countries (but mainly including flours, milk, and eggs), as well as cakes, doughnuts and other pastries (Anderson 2013).

Dairy products are also considered an important component of many traditional breakfasts. Yogurt is commonly consumed in India, and it is also present in Russia, the United States, and many countries in the Mediterranean region in Europe, North Africa, and the Levant. Cheeses are also widely consumed in Western countries, either with eggs or bread and even with fruits. Moreover, other remarkably essential items of breakfast meals are eggs. They can be served in a variety of ways, such as boiled, scrambled, fried, poached, cured, and as omelets, as well as used in recipes, like quiches, cakes, pastries, pancakes, *tortillas* and many more. On the other hand, meat products have not been an essential part of breakfast meals before the 19th century, since its consumption was restricted to wealthier people. With its increased accessibility over the years, cured meats such as bacon, ham, and sausages started to be included in breakfast meals in Europe and the United States.

Regarding seafood, its presence in traditional breakfast meals is seen in Jamaica and Japan. Besides fish, soups are also commonly consumed in Japan, as well as in other Asian countries, such as China and Vietnam. Lamb and Mutton stews, as well as fried rice, are also traditionally consumed in these countries (Anderson 2013).

Fruits, either fresh, as compotes, conserves, jams or juices, are also considered important items to compose a complete breakfast, especially in Western countries. At the same time, vegetables have been consumed for breakfast in the Middle East and the Levant, China, and Korea for centuries. Tea or coffee (pure or with added milk) are considered universal beverages consumed along with breakfast (Anderson 2013).

The International Breakfast Research Initiative analyzed the data of national nutrition surveys from six countries (Canada, Denmark, France, Spain, the UK, and the US) to establish general breakfast guidelines. In all countries, breakfast consisted mainly of a carbohydrate-rich and nutrient-dense meal, but also with sugar, sodium, and total fat intakes above the recommendations and low fiber intake. The study emphasizes the importance of establishing specific nutritional recommendations for breakfast to optimize strategies aimed at helping people to make healthier choices (Gibney et al. 2018). In France, for example, sweet breakfast (composed mainly by flavored milk, brioche, chocolate spread, and juice) was the most prevalent among 9-11 years old kids, and 83% of the participants consumed dairy products for breakfast (Lepicard et al. 2017). In Mexico, a study with 4-13 years old kids identified both traditional (composed by tortillas, beans, and eggs) and Westernized (composed by cereals and milk) meal patterns were identified (Afeiche et al. 2017). In the United States, foods commonly consumed by adults for breakfast include eggs, ready-to-eat cereals with milk, bread, coffee, and soft drinks, and high-fat desserts (Siega-Riz, Popkin, and Carson 2000).

A broad analysis of breakfast meals around the world shows that many of the items consumed fit into an ovo-lacto-vegetarian diet, with some minor exceptions (such as bacon, other cured meats, and, in a lower proportion, fish or chicken) (Anderson 2013). However, only a small portion of breakfast patterns would be suitable for vegans, since the consumption of eggs and milk is widely spread, either as a main dish (for example, omelet), added to meals (such as the milk or yogurt added to cereals) or as ingredients in recipes. Therefore, strict vegetarian meals need to be somehow adapted or prepared with other suitable components.

The dairy substitutes industry has been growing over the last years, as more consumers are looking for dairy alternatives. Not only strict vegetarians but also individuals with medical conditions, such as casein allergy or lactose intolerance (prevalent in 75% of the worldwide population), can benefit from the higher offer of plant-based milk substitutes (Mäkinen et al. 2016). These beverages are produced from legumes, seeds, cereals, and pseudocereals and have a similar aspect to cow's milk. In some aspects, they can be considered healthier substitutes, mainly due to its low saturated fat content, compared to cow's milk, as well as the presence of phytochemicals, which can bring cardiovascular protection. However, nutritional quality can be compromised during industrial production, mainly due to the addition of ingredients to increase stabilization, shelf-life, and improve palatability, such as sweeteners, oils, flavorings, salt, and stabilizers.

Moreover, nutritional values of plant milk can vary greatly, and they are usually lower in protein (except for legume-based drinks, such as soy or peanut milk), calcium, iodine, B12, B2, D and E vitamins, when compared to cow's milk. Some industrialized products might be fortified with these nutrients to resemble cow's milk composition. However, it is crucial to increase consumers' awareness about the differences in nutritional values among plant-based milk substitutes to adjust their diets to provide such nutrients from other sources, when necessary (Mäkinen et al. 2016). A particular concern is essential regarding kids since the intake of plant-based milk substitutes is not advised as a source of the above-cited nutrients (Verduci et al. 2019). Even though dairy products are not essential for humans, it is possible to obtain such nutrients from a plant-based diet. The high daily intake of plant-based milk, without the proper adjustment of the diet to guarantee the nutritional needs of the child, might pose them at a higher risk of nutrient deficiencies (Verduci et al. 2019). On the other hand, when diet quality is high, the intake of cow's milk is not necessary, it is unlikely to bring health benefits, and it could even increase the risk of fractures and some types of cancer later in life (Willett and Ludwig 2020).

BREAKFAST AND HEALTH EFFECTS

A cross-sectional study conducted in Germany correlated the breakfast quality with many health markers in the 668 participants (Iqbal et al. 2017). After adjustment for overall diet quality and other potential confounders, breakfast quality was positively associated with a better cardiometabolic profile. Eating industrialized foods for breakfast such as processed meat, margarine, sugar, and cheese was associated with a higher cardiometabolic risk score, glycated hemoglobin, triglycerides, diastolic blood pressure, waist circumference, and BMI, and lower HDL-c. On the other hand, a healthier eating pattern for breakfast (which included higher intake of cereals and tea) was inversely correlated to the cardiometabolic risk score, glycated hemoglobin, and BMI, and positively correlated with HDL-c. Better breakfast quality was also positively associated with higher calorie intake for breakfast (Iqbal et al. 2017).

These results are in line with evidence showing that whole-grain intake is associated with reduced risk of cardiovascular diseases, cancer, and all-cause mortality, as well as type 2 diabetes, obesity, and weight gain (Aune et al. 2016; Ye et al. 2012). Nonetheless, processed meats are associated with increased mortality (Wang et al. 2016). Reduced intake of saturated fat (which comes mainly from animal sources), and trans fat (industrially produced from vegetable oil hydrogenation) can bring health benefits (Nettleton et al. 2017; Wang et al. 2016). Therefore, including whole-grain cereals such as oats and whole-grain bread and at the same time reducing processed meats, margarine, and other industrialized foods for breakfast can bring many health benefits.

Especially among western countries, low-quality meals, mainly based on refined carbohydrates, and saturated fat, are commonly eaten, correlating with increased risk of chronic diseases. Examples of unhealthy foods widely consumed for breakfast include sugary breakfast cereals, white bread with butter, margarine or jam, cakes, pancakes, waffles, and sugary drinks (milk chocolate, sweetened coffee, or tea, artificial juices). The high intake of sugar and refined carbohydrates can lead to impaired glucose metabolism, increased inflammatory markers, and weight gain (Spreadbury 2012; Aeberli et al. 2011; Morenga, Mallard, and Mann 2013). Therefore, over the last years, health professionals, studies, and media have put effort into encouraging a reduction of refined carbohydrates to promote health improvement.

On the other hand, claiming that carbohydrates are detrimental to health might give the wrong interpretation that all types and sources of carbohydrates have the same effect on the body. Contrary to sugar and refined sources such as white flours, whole foods (such as fruits, vegetables, and grains, which also contain a high carbohydrate content) are linked to better health parameters and lower risk of chronic diseases and mortality (Temple 2018; Reynolds et al. 2019; Aune et al. 2016).

However, due to the growing trend of carbohydrate avoidance, "low carb" diets have gained space in the media, with their defenders claiming that eating food higher in fat and protein and lower in carbohydrates would bring more health benefits. Indeed, studies have already shown that higher protein meals can bring some benefits, such as lower ghrelin levels (resulting in more satiety) and lower post-prandial glycemic peaks. Therefore, a higher protein diet can be considered a good strategy for weight loss (Halton and Hu 2004; Roberts et al. 2019; Westerterp-Plantenga et al. 2009; Dhillon et al. 2016). Nonetheless, most studies that evaluate the effects of protein intake are short-term and do not take into account the protein sources (animal versus plants) or the potentially harmful long-term effects of eating a higher protein diet on health and longevity. The protein source is relevant because animal protein intake has been linked to a lower life span, while vegetable protein does not seem to affect longevity (Brandhorst and Longo 2019). Moreover, it has already been described that high protein intake, especially when it comes from animal sources, can lead to poorer health, inducing cellular signaling related to impaired insulin response, increased inflammation, aging, and mortality (Kitada et al. 2019; Mirzaei, Suarez, and Longo 2014; Azemati et al. 2017). However, eating more protein is still considered a "health goal." People are often worried about not getting enough protein, even though a Western diet easily exceeds the protein recommendations (US Department of Agriculture; Agricultural Research Service 2009; Sans and Combris 2015; Rippin et al. 2017).

When it comes to breakfast, this "low carb" trend shifted the recommendations towards more animal-based high-fat meals, which include eggs, bacon, cheese, and even coffee with butter (bulletproof coffee). Despite the potential benefits of satiety, a single high saturated fat meal can increase inflammatory markers over the following hours (Herieka and Erridge 2014). If this meal pattern is maintained daily, with the inclusion of breakfast based on animal products, this could potentially lead to an increased risk of non-communicable diseases and mortality. Therefore, including unrefined plant-based foods for breakfast is an excellent strategy to promote more satiety but avoid the harmful health effects of excess animal-foods intake. Vegetable protein sources are considered even more satiating than animal sources (Kristensen et al. 2016). Moreover, plant-based foods rich in fiber can contribute to satiety and lower food intake throughout the day, since fibers can reach the gut and induce the production of GLP-1. This important mechanism controls food intake due to its anorexigenic effect (Sleeth et al. 2010).

A higher intake of fiber also promotes better gut health with a more balanced microbiome. Fibers are also fermented into short-chain fatty acids, which, in turn, reduce inflammation in the gut and systemically, contribute to the prevention and control of chronic diseases (Makki et al. 2018). On the other hand, higher protein intake can harm the gut microbiome, stimulating the production of potentially toxic compounds by the microbiota. Such a detrimental effect is counterbalanced by adding fiber to a high protein meal (Diether and Willing 2019), which reinforces the need to include good fiber sources to a breakfast meal, mainly when composed of animal-protein sources, which are absent in fiber. Therefore, a moderate protein meal, comprising mostly vegetable protein sources, as well as rich in fiber, could have all the satiety effects of a high animal protein meal without the potentially harmful effect of a high animal protein consumption in the long term.

PLANT-BASED BREAKFAST ALTERNATIVES

Plant-based breakfast meals can be composed of a wide range of items to provide adequate nutrients intake and also guarantee desirable sensorial features. Fruits, vegetables, cereals, legumes, nuts, and seeds can be used for this purpose. Combining different food groups into meals and preparations, as well as substituting typical omnivore or ovolactovegetarian ingredients for plant-based foods, can also provide similar meals. It is still aligned with the individuals' preferences, since many people exclude animal products from their diet due to ethical, environmental or religious reasons (D. E. Slywitch 2015), but might still enjoy their taste.

Fruits can be eaten raw or used in smoothies, baked goods (such as cakes, cookies, bread) to add flavor and sweetness, as well as consumed with cereals (oats, granola), porridges and as blended fruit creams. Green juices or smoothies are also an easy way to include fruits and vegetables to the breakfast meal.

Vegetables, especially the dark green ones, can be included to breakfast meals to provide essential nutrients such as calcium, iron, magnesium, potassium, as well as carotenoids, fiber, phytochemicals, carotenoids, and B vitamins (Colonna et al. 2016; Liu 2013; Amagloh et al. 2017). Since vegetables are not commonly consumed in breakfast among most Western countries, a good alternative would be to include them in bread preparations, rice bowls, or soups, which are typical breakfast options in Mediterranean and Asian countries (Anderson 2013).

Cereals are commonly eaten all over the world on a breakfast basis. Porridges can be prepared with water or plant-based milk substitutes, with fruits or dried fruits (when eaten sweet), or with vegetable broth instead of beef broth (when made in the savory version). Bread, a widely consumed breakfast item, is usually made only with plant-based ingredients. However, as some recipes might include eggs or dairy, consumers' awareness about the bread composition is important to suit their dietary restrictions. In Asian countries, rice is also a critical breakfast item, which can be consumed with vegetables and legumes to provide a more nutritious meal (Murakami, Livingstone, and Sasaki 2017; Tan et al. 2018).

Legumes are considered an essential source of protein, vitamins, and minerals, as well as fibers and phytochemicals, in vegetarian diets (Erbersdobler, Barth, and Jahreis 2017). In Mexico, for example, bean tortillas are commonly consumed for breakfast. Hummus, a chickpea-based paste, can be eaten with bread as a substitute for dairy spreads, such as creamy cheeses. Tofu, a soy-based cheese substitute, can also be eaten with bread, or as an egg substitute (in a scrambled form), since it is high in protein (Baines 2013) and can have similar sensorial features. Moreover, legumes can be added to rice bowls and soups, and even fruit smoothies, to add nutritional value. Plant-based milk made from legumes can also provide more nutrients than cereal-based milk substitutes and are more versatile in typical Western breakfast meals, such as cereals with milk.

Nuts and seeds can be included in a vegetarian breakfast to provide good sources of unsaturated fats, fibers, protein, and other essential nutrients (De Souza et al. 2017). They can be added to fruit bowls, porridges, and smoothies, either in their natural form or as spreads. Peanuts, from the legumes group, are also included in this category due to their nutritional similarity. Peanut and nuts kinds of butter are good spread substitutes in bread. Tahini, a sesame paste typically consumed in Arabic countries, is a good source of calcium (Mangels 2014), and it can also be eaten with bread or as an ingredient to hummus, different sauces, and even smoothies. Almond and other nuts' milk are also gaining popularity and can easily be added into recipes and beverages.

Plant-based breakfast alternatives should not be based on highly refined and industrialized foods. Many options such as vegan milk, cheeses, cakes, industrialized bread, cookies, pastries, and breakfast cereals can be loaded with added sugar, refined oils, excess of food additives and sodium, as well as have a low nutritional value. Therefore, a whole foods plant-based breakfast, based on natural unrefined foods, must be encouraged to guarantee all the benefits associated with a healthy vegetarian dietary pattern.

CONCLUSION

Due to all the described benefits of eating breakfast, stimulating its consumption, as well as a higher caloric intake during the morning period compared to night time, is a vital strategy to help control chronic diseases. However, more emphasis should be given to the meal quality since specific food choices might have detrimental effects on health. Fruits, vegetables, whole carbohydrates options, and protein-rich beverages are good options to improve vegetarian breakfasts. When looking for industrialized versions, always look carefully at their labels. The list of ingredients shows if animal products or byproducts were used, and the type of feedstock.

Having a breakfast meal rich in non-processed plant-based foods might contribute to a better outcome, when compared to an animal-based meal, considering all the potential benefits that plant-based diets have over animal foods for health on a long-term.

REFERENCES

Academy of Nutrition and Dietetics. 2016. "Position of the Academy of Nutrition and Dietetics: Vegetarian Diets." *Journal of the Academy of Nutrition and Dietetics* 116 (12): 1970–80. https://doi.org/10.1016/j.jand.2016.09.025.

Aeberli, Isabelle, Philipp A. Gerber, Michel Hochuli, Sibylle Kohler, Sarah R. Haile, Ioanna Gouni-Berthold, Heiner K. Berthold, Giatgen A. Spinas, and Kaspar Berneis. 2011. "Low to Moderate Sugar-Sweetened Beverage Consumption Impairs Glucose and Lipid Metabolism and Promotes Inflammation in Healthy Young Men: A Randomized Controlled Trial." *American Journal of Clinical Nutrition* 94 (2): 479–85. https://doi.org/10.3945/ajcn.111.013540.

Afeiche, Myriam C, Lindsey Smith Taillie, Sinead Hopkins, Alison L Eldridge, and Barry M Popkin. 2017. "Breakfast Dietary Patterns among Mexican Children Are Related to Total-Day Diet Quality." *The Journal of Nutrition*, no. C: jn239780. https://doi.org/10.3945/jn.116.239780.

Afshin, Ashkan, Mohammad H. Forouzanfar, Marissa B. Reitsma, Patrick Sur, Kara Estep, Alex Lee, Laurie Marczak, et al. 2017. "Health Effects of Overweight and Obesity in 195 Countries over 25 Years." *New England Journal of Medicine* 377 (1): 13–27. https://doi.org/10.1056/NEJMoa1614362.

Amagloh, Francis, Richard Atuna, Richard McBride, Edward Carey, and Tatiana Christides. 2017. "Nutrient and Total Polyphenol Contents of Dark Green Leafy Vegetables, and Estimation of Their Iron

Bioaccessibility Using the In Vitro Digestion/Caco-2 Cell Model." *Foods* 6 (7): 54. https://doi.org/10.3390/foods6070054.

Anderson, Heather Arndt. 2013. *Breakfast: A History*. Edited by Ken Albala. 1st ed. AltaMira Press.

Aune, Dagfinn, NaNa Keum, Edward Giovannucci, Lars T. Fadnes, Paolo Boffetta, Darren C. Greenwood, Serena Tonstad, Lars J. Vatten, Elio Riboli, and Teresa Norat. 2016. "Whole Grain Consumption and Risk of Cardiovascular Disease, Cancer, and All Cause and Cause Specific Mortality: Systematic Review and Dose-Response Meta-Analysis of Prospective Studies." *BMJ* 353 (2716): 1–14. https://doi.org/10.1136/bmj.i2716.

Azemati, Bahar, Sujatha Rajaram, Karen Jaceldo-Siegl, Joan Sabate, David Shavlik, Gary E Fraser, and Ella H Haddad. 2017. "Animal-Protein Intake Is Associated with Insulin Resistance in Adventist Health Study 2 (AHS-2) Calibration Substudy Participants: A Cross-Sectional Analysis." *Current Developments in Nutrition* 1 (4): e000299. https://doi.org/10.3945/cdn.116.000299.

Baines, Surinder K. 2013. "Protein and Vegetarian Diets." *The Medical Journal of Australia* 199 (4): S7–10. https://doi.org/10.5694/mjao11.11492.

Ballon, Aurélie, Manuela Neuenschwander, and Sabrina Schlesinger. 2018. "Breakfast Skipping Is Associated with Increased Risk of Type 2 Diabetes among Adults: A Systematic Review and Meta-Analysis of Prospective Cohort Studies," 1–8.

Barbaresko, Janett, Manja Koch, Matthias B. Schulze, and Ute Nöthlings. 2013. "Dietary Pattern Analysis and Biomarkers of Low-Grade Inflammation: A Systematic Literature Review." *Nutrition Reviews* 71 (8): 511–27. https://doi.org/10.1111/nure.12035.

Bi, Huashan, Yong Gan, Chen Yang, Yawen Chen, Xinyue Tong, and Zuxun Lu. 2015. "Breakfast Skipping and the Risk of Type 2 Diabetes: A Meta-Analysis of Observational Studies." *Public Health Nutrition* 18 (16): 3013–19. https://doi.org/10.1017/S1368980015000257.

Bradbury, K. E., F. L. Crowe, P. N. Appleby, J. A. Schmidt, R. C. Travis, and T. J. Key. 2014. "Serum Concentrations of Cholesterol,

Apolipoprotein A-I and Apolipoprotein B in a Total of 1694 Meat-Eaters, Fish-Eaters, Vegetarians and Vegans." *European Journal of Clinical Nutrition* 68 (2): 178–83. https://doi.org/10.1038/ejcn. 2013.248.

Brandhorst, Sebastian, and Valter D. Longo. 2019. "Protein Quantity and Source, Fasting-Mimicking Diets, and Longevity." *Advances in Nutrition (Bethesda, Md.)* 10 (4): S340–50. https://doi.org/10.1093/advances/nmz079.

Chen, X. U. E., Renata Pyzik, Angie Yong, and Gary E. Striker. 2010. "Advanced Glycation End Products in Foods and a Practical Guide to Their Reduction in the Diet." *Journal of the American Dietetic Association* 110 (6): 911–16. https://doi.org/10.1016/j.jada.2010. 03.018.Advanced.

Chiu, Tina H. T., Wen Harn Pan, Ming Nan Lin, and Chin Lon Lin. 2018. "Vegetarian Diet, Change in Dietary Patterns, and Diabetes Risk: A Prospective Study." *Nutrition and Diabetes* 8 (1). https://doi.org/10. 1038/s41387-018-0022-4.

Clarys, Peter, Tom Deliens, Inge Huybrechts, Peter Deriemaeker, Barbara Vanaelst, Willem De Keyzer, Marcel Hebbelinck, and Patrick Mullie. 2014. "Comparison of Nutritional Quality of the Vegan, Vegetarian, Semi-Vegetarian, Pesco-Vegetarian and Omnivorous Diet." *Nutrients* 6 (3): 1318–32. https://doi.org/10.3390/nu6031318.

Colonna, Emma, Youssef Rouphael, Giancarlo Barbieri, and Stefania De Pascale. 2016. "Nutritional Quality of Ten Leafy Vegetables Harvested at Two Light Intensities." *Food Chemistry* 199: 702–10. https://doi.org/10.1016/j.foodchem.2015.12.068.

Dhillon, Jaapna, Bruce A. Craig, Heather J. Leidy, Akua F. Amankwaah, Katherene Osei-Boadi Anguah, Ashley Jacobs, Blake L. Jones, et al. 2016. "The Effects of Increased Protein Intake on Fullness: A Meta-Analysis and Its Limitations." *Journal of the Academy of Nutrition and Dietetics* 116 (6): 968–83. https://doi.org/10.1016/j.jand.2016.01.003.

Diether, Natalie E., and Benjamin P. Willing. 2019. "Microbial Fermentation of Dietary Protein: An Important Factor in Diet–Microbe–

Host Interaction." *Microorganisms* 7 (1). https://doi.org/10.3390/microorganisms7010019.

Erbersdobler, Helmut F, Christian A Barth, and Gerhard Jahreis. 2017. "Legumes in Human Nutrition: Nutrient Content and Protein Quality of Pulses Fatty Acid Distribution." *Science & Research | Overview 140 Ernaehrungs Umschau International* 10 (October). https://doi.org/10.4455/eu.2017.038.

Gibney, Michael J., Susan I. Barr, France Bellisle, Adam Drewnowski, Sisse Fagt, Sinead Hopkins, Barbara Livingstone, et al. 2018. "Towards an Evidence-Based Recommendation for a Balanced Breakfast—A Proposal from the International Breakfast Research Initiative." *Nutrients* 10 (10). https://doi.org/10.3390/nu10101540.

Halton, Thomas L, and Frank B Hu. 2004. "The Effects of High Protein Diets on Thermogenesis, Satiety and Weight Loss: A Critical Review." *Journal of the American College of Nutrition* 23 (5).

Henry, Christiani Jeyakumar, Bhupinder Kaur, and Rina Yu Chin Quek. 2020. "Chrononutrition in the Management of Diabetes." *Nutrition and Diabetes* 10 (1). https://doi.org/10.1038/s41387-020-0109-6.

Herieka, Mohammed, and Clett Erridge. 2014. "High-Fat Meal Induced Postprandial Inflammation." *Molecular Nutrition and Food Research* 58 (1): 136–46. https://doi.org/10.1002/mnfr.201300104.

Inteligência, IBOPE. 2018. *14% Da População Se Declara Vegetariana.* 2018. [*14% of the population declares itself to be vegetarian.*]

Iqbal, K., L. Schwingshackl, M. Gottschald, S. Knüppel, M. Stelmach-Mardas, K. Aleksandrova, and H. Boeing. 2017. "Breakfast Quality and Cardiometabolic Risk Profiles in an Upper Middle-Aged German Population." *European Journal of Clinical Nutrition* 71 (11): 1312–20. https://doi.org/10.1038/ejcn.2017.116.

Kahleova, H., M. Matoulek, H. Malinska, O. Oliyarnik, L. Kazdova, T. Neskudla, A. Skoch, et al. 2011. "Vegetarian Diet Improves Insulin Resistance and Oxidative Stress Markers More than Conventional Diet in Subjects with Type2 Diabetes." *Diabetic Medicine* 28 (5): 549–59. https://doi.org/10.1111/j.1464-5491.2010.03209.x.

Kahleova, H., and T. Pelikanova. 2015. "Vegetarian Diets in the Prevention and Treatment of Type 2 Diabetes." *Journal of the American College of Nutrition* 34 (5): 1–11. https://doi.org/10.1080/07315724.2014.976890.

Kahleova, Hana, Rebecca Fleeman, Adela Hlozkova, Richard Holubkov, and Neal D. Barnard. 2018. "A Plant-Based Diet in Overweight Individuals in a 16-Week Randomized Clinical Trial: Metabolic Benefits of Plant Protein." *Nutrition and Diabetes* 8 (1). https://doi.org/10.1038/s41387-018-0067-4.

Kahleova, Hana, Susan Levin, and Neal D. Barnard. 2018. "Vegetarian Dietary Patterns and Cardiovascular Disease." *Progress in Cardiovascular Diseases* 61 (1): 54–61. https://doi.org/10.1016/j.pcad.2018.05.002.

Kessler, Katharina, and Olga Pivovarova-Ramich. 2019. "Meal Timing, Aging, and Metabolic Health." *International Journal of Molecular Sciences* 20 (8): 1–16. https://doi.org/10.3390/ijms20081911.

Kim, Mi Kyung, Sang Woon Cho, and Yoo Kyoung Park. 2012. "Long-Term Vegetarians Have Low Oxidative Stress, Body Fat, and Cholesterol Levels." *Nutrition Research and Practice* 6 (2): 155–61. https://doi.org/10.4162/nrp.2012.6.2.155.

Kitada, Munehiro, Yoshio Ogura, Itaru Monno, and Daisuke Koya. 2019. "The Impact of Dietary Protein Intake on Longevity and Metabolic Health." *EBioMedicine* 43: 632–40. https://doi.org/10.1016/j.ebiom.2019.04.005.

Koeth, Robert a, Zeneng Wang, Bruce S Levison, Jennifer a Buffa, Elin Org, Brendan T Sheehy, Earl B Britt, et al. 2013. "Intestinal Microbiota Metabolism of L-Carnitine, a Nutrient in Red Meat, Promotes Atherosclerosis." *Nat Med* 19 (5): 576–85. https://doi.org/10.1038/nm.3145.Intestinal.

Kristensen, Marlene D., Nathalie T. Bendsen, Sheena M. Christensen, Arne Astrup, and Anne Raben. 2016. "Meals Based on Vegetable Protein Sources (Beans and Peas) Are More Satiating than Meals Based on Animal Protein Sources (Veal and Pork) - A Randomized Cross-over Meal Test Study." *Food and Nutrition Research* 60: 1–9. https://doi.org/10.3402/fnr.v60.32634.

Lepicard, E. M., M. Maillot, F. Vieux, M. Viltard, and F. Bonnet. 2017. "Quantitative and Qualitative Analysis of Breakfast Nutritional Composition in French Schoolchildren Aged 9–11 Years." *Journal of Human Nutrition and Dietetics* 30 (2): 151–58. https://doi.org/10.1111/jhn.12412.

Liu, Rui Hai. 2013. "Health-Promoting Components of Fruits and Vegetables in the Diet." *Advances in Nutrition* 4: 384S–392S. https://doi.org/10.3945/an.112.003517.convenient.

Mäkinen, Outi Elina, Viivi Wanhalinna, Emanuele Zannini, and Elke Karin Arendt. 2016. "Foods for Special Dietary Needs: Non-Dairy Plant-Based Milk Substitutes and Fermented Dairy-Type Products." *Critical Reviews in Food Science and Nutrition* 56 (3): 339–49. https://doi.org/10.1080/10408398.2012.761950.

Makki, Kassem, Edward C. Deehan, Jens Walter, and Fredrik Bäckhed. 2018. "The Impact of Dietary Fiber on Gut Microbiota in Host Health and Disease." *Cell Host and Microbe* 23 (6): 705–15. https://doi.org/10.1016/j.chom.2018.05.012.

Mangels, Ann Reed. 2014. "Bone Nutrients for Vegetarians." *American Journal of Clinical Nutrition* 100 (SUPPL. 1). https://doi.org/10.3945/ajcn.113.071423.

McEvoy, Claire T., and Jayne V. Woodside. 2015. "2.9 Vegetarian Diets." In *Pediatric Nutrition in Practice*, edited by B. (Munich) Koletzko, GA) Bhatia, J. (Augusta, Z. A. (Karachi) Bhutta, P. (Johannesburg) Cooper, SA) Makrides, M. (Adelaide, R. (Santiago de Chile) Uauy, and W. (Shanghai) Wang, 113:134–38. Basel, Switzerland: karger. https://doi.org/10.1159/000367873.

Mirzaei, Hamed, Jorge A. Suarez, and Valter D. Longo. 2014. "Protein and Amino Acid Restriction, Aging and Disease: From Yeast to Humans." *Trends Endocrinol Metab* 25 (11): 558–66. https://doi.org/10.1038/jid.2014.371.

Moore, Wendy J., Michael E. McGrievy, and Gabrielle M. Turner-McGrievy. 2015. "Dietary Adherence and Acceptability of Five Different Diets, Including Vegan and Vegetarian Diets, for Weight

Loss: The New DIETs Study." *Eating Behaviors* 19: 33–38. https://doi.org/10.1016/j.eatbeh.2015.06.011.

Morenga, Lisa Te, Simonette Mallard, and Jim Mann. 2013. "Dietary Sugars and Body Weight: Systematic Review and Meta-Analyses of Randomised Controlled Trials and Cohort Studies." *BMJ (Online)* 345 (7891): 1–25. https://doi.org/10.1136/bmj.e7492.

Murakami, Kentaro, M. Barbara E. Livingstone, and Satoshi Sasaki. 2017. "Establishment of a Meal Coding System for the Characterization of Meal-Based Dietary Patterns in Japan." *The Journal of Nutrition*, no. C: jn254896. https://doi.org/10.3945/jn.117.254896.

Najjar, Rami S., Carolyn E. Moore, and Baxter D. Montgomery. 2018. "Consumption of a Defined, Plant-Based Diet Reduces Lipoprotein(a), Inflammation, and Other Atherogenic Lipoproteins and Particles within 4 Weeks." *Clinical Cardiology* 41 (8): 1062–68. https://doi.org/10.1002/clc.23027.

Nettleton, Joyce A., Ingeborg A. Brouwer, Johanna M. Geleijnse, and Gerard Hornstra. 2017. "Saturated Fat Consumption and Risk of Coronary Heart Disease and Ischemic Stroke: A Science Update." *Annals of Nutrition and Metabolism* 70 (1): 26–33. https://doi.org/10.1159/000455681.

Orlich, Michael J., and Gary E. Fraser. 2014. "Vegetarian Diets in the Adventist Health Study 2: A Review of Initial Published Findings." *American Journal of Clinical Nutrition* 100 ((suppl)): 353S-8S. https://doi.org/10.3945/ajcn.113.071233.Am.

Oussalah, Abderrahim, Julien Levy, Clémence Berthezène, David H. Alpers, and Jean Louis Guéant. 2020. "Health Outcomes Associated with Vegetarian Diets: An Umbrella Review of Systematic Reviews and Meta-Analyses." *Clinical Nutrition*. https://doi.org/10.1016/j.clnu.2020.02.037.

Reynolds, Andrew, Jim Mann, John Cummings, Nicola Winter, Evelyn Mete, and Lisa Te Morenga. 2019. "Carbohydrate Quality and Human Health: A Series of Systematic Reviews and Meta-Analyses." *The Lancet* 393 (10170): 434–45. https://doi.org/10.1016/S0140-6736(18)31809-9.

Rippin, Holly L., Jayne Hutchinson, Jo Jewell, Joao J. Breda, and Janet E. Cade. 2017. "Adult Nutrient Intakes from Current National Dietary Surveys of European Populations." *Nutrients* 9 (12): 1–47. https://doi.org/10.3390/nu9121288.

Roberts, Justin, Anastasia Zinchenko, Krishnaa Mahbubani, James Johnstone, Lee Smith, Viviane Merzbach, Miguel Blacutt, et al. 2019. "Satiating Effect of High Protein Diets on Resistance-Trained Subjects in Energy Deficit." *Nutrients* 11 (1): 1–21. https://doi.org/10.3390/nu11010056.

Sans, P., and P. Combris. 2015. "World Meat Consumption Patterns: An Overview of the Last Fifty Years (1961-2011)." *Meat Science* 109: 106–11. https://doi.org/10.1016/j.meatsci.2015.05.012.

Satija, Ambika, Shilpa N. Bhupathiraju, Eric B. Rimm, Donna Spiegelman, Stephanie E. Chiuve, Lea Borgi, Walter C. Willett, Jo Ann E. Manson, Qi Sun, and Frank B. Hu. 2016. "Plant-Based Dietary Patterns and Incidence of Type 2 Diabetes in US Men and Women: Results from Three Prospective Cohort Studies." *PLoS Medicine* 13 (6). https://doi.org/10.1371/journal.pmed.1002039.

Shi, Hang, Huali Yin, Jeffrey S. Flier, Hang Shi, Maia V. Kokoeva, Karen Inouye, Iphigenia Tzameli, Huali Yin, and Jeffrey S. Flier. 2006. "TLR4 Links Innate Immunity and Fatty Acid – Induced Insulin Resistance Find the Latest Version: TLR4 Links Innate Immunity and Fatty Acid – Induced Insulin Resistance." *The Journal of Clinical Investigation* 116 (11): 3015–25. https://doi.org/10.1172/JCI28898.TLRs.

Siega-Riz, Anna Maria, Barry M. Popkin, and Terri Carson. 2000. "Differences in Food Patterns at Breakfast by Sociodemographic Characteristics among a Nationally Representative Sample of Adults in the United States." *Preventive Medicine* 30 (5): 415–24. https://doi.org/10.1006/pmed.2000.0651.

Sleeth, Michelle L., Emily L. Thompson, Heather E. Ford, Sagen E. K. Zac-Varghese, and Gary Frost. 2010. "Free Fatty Acid Receptor 2 and Nutrient Sensing: A Proposed Role for Fibre, Fermentable Carbohydrates and Short-Chain Fatty Acids in Appetite Regulation."

Nutrition Research Reviews 23 (1): 135–45. https://doi.org/10.1017/S0954422410000089.

Sluijs, Ivonne, Joline W. J. Beulens, Daphne L. Van Der A, Annemieke M. W. Spijkerman, Diederick E. Grobbee, and Yvonne T. Van Der Schouw. 2010. "Dietary Intake of Total, Animal, and Vegetable Protein and Risk of Type 2 Diabetes in the European Prospective Investigation into Cancer and Nutrition (EPIC)-NL Study." *Diabetes Care* 33 (1): 43–48. https://doi.org/10.2337/dc09-1321.

Slywitch, Dr. Eric. 2015. *Alimentação Sem Carne - Um Guia Prático Para Montar a Sua Dieta Vegetariana Com Saúde*. Edited by Alaúde Editorial LTDA. 2a Edição. São Paulo: Alaúde Editorial LTDA. [*Meatless Eating - A Practical Guide To Setting Up Your Healthy Vegetarian Diet.*]

Slywitch, Eric. 2012. *Guia Alimentar de Dietas Vegetarianas*. Edited by Departamento de Medicina e Nutrição - Sociedade Vegetariana Brasileira. Sociedade Vegetariana Brasileira. São Paulo, Brasil. [*Food Guide for Vegetarian Diets.*]

Souza, Rávila Graziany Machado De, Raquel Machado Schincaglia, Gustavo Duarte Pimente, and João Felipe Mota. 2017. "Nuts and Human Health Outcomes: A Systematic Review." *Nutrients* 9 (12). https://doi.org/10.3390/nu9121311.

Spencer, E. A., P. N. Appleby, G. K. Davey, and T. J. Key. 2003. "Diet and Body Mass Index in 38 000 EPIC-Oxford Meat-Eaters, Fish-Eaters, Vegetarians and Vegans." *International Journal of Obesity* 27: 728–34. https://doi.org/10.1038/sj.ijo.0802300.

Spreadbury, Ian. 2012. *Comparison with Ancestral Diets Suggests Dense Acellular Carbohydrates Promote an Inflammatory Microbiota, and May Be the Primary Dietary Cause of Leptin Resistance and Obesity*, 175–89.

Statista. 2016. "Vegetarian Diet Followers Worldwide by Region." 2016.

Tan, Wei Shuan Kimberly, Wei Jie Kevin Tan, Shalini D.O. Ponnalagu, Katie Koecher, Ravi Menon, Sze Yen Tan, and Christiani J. Henry. 2018. "The Glycaemic Index and Insulinaemic Index of Commercially Available Breakfast and Snack Foods in an Asian Population." *British*

Journal of Nutrition 119 (10): 1151–56. https://doi.org/10.1017/S0007 114518000703.

Temple, Norman J. 2018. "Fat, Sugar, Whole Grains and Heart Disease: 50 Years of Confusion." *Nutrients* 10 (1): 1–9. https://doi.org/10.3390/nu10010039.

Touvier, Mathilde, Julia Baudry, Sandrine Péneau, Emmanuelle Kesse-Guyot, Serge Hercberg, Caroline Méjean, and Benjamin Allès. 2017. "Comparison of Sociodemographic and Nutritional Characteristics between Self-Reported Vegetarians, Vegans, and Meat-Eaters from the NutriNet-Santé Study." *Nutrients* 9 (9): 1023. https://doi.org/10.3390/nu9091023.

US Department of Agriculture; Agricultural Research Service. 2009. "What We Eat in America: Nutrient Intakes from Food by Gender and Age." *National Health and Nutrition Examination Survey (NHANES) 2009-10*.

Uzhova, Irina, Valentín Fuster, Antonio Fernández-Ortiz, José M. Ordovás, Javier Sanz, Leticia Fernández-Friera, Beatriz López-Melgar, et al. 2017. "The Importance of Breakfast in Atherosclerosis Disease: Insights From the PESA Study." *Journal of the American College of Cardiology* 70 (15): 1833–42. https://doi.org/10.1016/j.jacc.2017.08.027.

Verduci, Elvira, Sofia D'elios, Lucia Cerrato, Pasquale Comberiati, Mauro Calvani, Samuele Palazzo, Alberto Martelli, Massimo Landi, Thulja Trikamjee, and Diego G. Peroni. 2019. "Cow's Milk Substitutes for Children: Nutritional Aspects of Milk from Different Mammalian Species, Special Formula and Plant-Based Beverages." *Nutrients* 11 (8): 3–4. https://doi.org/10.3390/nu11081739.

Wang, Dong D, Yanping Li, Stephanie E Chiuve, Meir J Stampfer, Joann E Manson, Eric B Rimm, Walter C Willett, and Frank B Hu. 2016. "Specific Dietary Fats in Relation to Total and Cause-Specific Mortality HHS Public Access." *JAMA Intern Med* 176 (8): 1134–45. https://doi.org/10.1001/jamainternmed.2016.2417.

Wang, Xia, Xinying Lin, Ying Y. Ouyang, Jun Liu, Gang Zhao, An Pan, and Frank B. Hu. 2016. "Red and Processed Meat Consumption and Mortality: Dose-Response Meta-Analysis of Prospective Cohort

Studies." *Public Health Nutrition* 19 (5): 893–905. https://doi.org/10.1017/S1368980015002062.

Westerterp-Plantenga, M. S., A. Nieuwenhuizen, D. Tomé, S. Soenen, and K.R. Westerterp. 2009. "Dietary Protein, Weight Loss, and Weight Maintenance." *Annual Review of Nutrition* 29 (1): 21–41. https://doi.org/10.1146/annurev-nutr-080508-141056.

Willett, Walter C., and David S. Ludwig. 2020. "Milk and Health." *The New England Journal of Medicine* 19 (1): 644–54. https://doi.org/10.1111/j.1471-0307.1966.tb01811.x.

Ye, Eva Qing, Sara A. Chacko, Elizabeth L. Chou, Matthew Kugizaki, and Simin Liu. 2012. "Greater Whole-Grain Intake Is Associated with Lower Risk of Type 2 Diabetes, Cardiovascular Disease, and Weight Gain." *The Journal of Nutrition* 142 (7): 1304–13. https://doi.org/10.3945/jn.111.155325.

Yokoyama, Yoko, Kunihiro Nishimura, Neal D. Barnard, Misa Takegami, Makoto Watanabe, Akira Sekikawa, Tomonori Okamura, and Yoshihiro Miyamoto. 2014. "Vegetarian Diets and Blood Pressure." *JAMA Intern Med*.

Zhao, Zhuoxian, Sheyu Li, Guanjian Liu, Fangfang Yan, Xuelei Ma, Zeyu Huang, and Haoming Tian. 2012. "Body Iron Stores and Heme-Iron Intake in Relation to Risk of Type 2 Diabetes: A Systematic Review and Meta-Analysis." *PLoS ONE* 7 (7). https://doi.org/10.1371/journal.pone.0041641.

In: Breakfast
Editor: Petr Měchura

ISBN: 978-1-53618-500-3
© 2020 Nova Science Publishers, Inc.

Chapter 3

GLUTEN-CONTAINING PRODUCTS IN BREAKFAST AND THEIR SUBSTITUTES IN GLUTEN-RELATED DISORDERS

Renata Puppin Zandonadi[*]
and Raquel Braz Assunção Botelho
Department of Nutrition, University of Brasília,
Brasília, DF, Brazil

ABSTRACT

The adverse reactions to gluten-containing products are increasing worldwide. Gluten-related disorders (GRD) include celiac disease, non-celiac gluten sensitivity, gluten ataxia, gluten, or wheat allergy, among others, reaching almost 10% of the worldwide population following the gluten-free diet (GFD). Breakfast is one of the meals that present a high consumption of gluten-containing foods (bread, cake, pancake, waffle, cereals, cookies, crackers, etc.). Breakfast is described as one of the most important meals of the day, generally consumed before going to work and reaching close to 20% of the nutritional recommendations. Therefore, it is

---

[*] Corresponding Author's E-mail: renatapz@yahoo.com.br.

a challenge to substitute gluten-containing products in breakfast due to the population's habit of consumption, the lack of gluten-free with nutritional, sensory, and technological quality, the cost of the substitutes, among others. In this context, the evaluation of breakfast gluten-containing products and their counterparts without gluten is important to help people with GRD to adequate their diet and to reduce the psychological burden of GFD.

Keywords: gluten, breakfast, gluten-related disorders, gluten-free

INTRODUCTION

Gluten, a water-insoluble protein complex, is available in some kinds of cereals (wheat, barley, oats, and rye) [1, 2]. Such a complex constitutes a network of proteins composed of the prolamin fractions of cereal-grains (gliadin, secalin, hordein, and avenin) and glutenin [2, 3]. Although some studies have established that oats are a safe cereal for most celiacs, some studies emphasize that their prolamin fraction, avenin, exerts toxicity in a subgroup of celiacs. It is also noteworthy the difficulty in guaranteeing oats production without cross-contamination by other cereals with gluten and, therefore, their consumption is discouraged in some countries for individuals with gluten-related disorders (GRD) [4–6]. However, since oats present avenin (prolamin) and glutenin, they are capable of forming the gluten chain, despite in most cases they are non-toxic to GRD individuals.

The use of gluten in the industry and the production of food at home or restaurants is vast, given its plurality of rheological characteristics [7, 8]. In contact with water, the gluten-complex produces a viscoelastic mass capable of elongating, deforming, and recovering its shape, as well as retaining gases, providing mass growth [7]. Therefore, it is widely used in the production of pasta, cookies, sauces, breaded, and as a thickening agent in ready to eat food [7–9].

Gluten-containing products are widely consumed worldwide, mainly through foods produced using wheat flour [10, 11]. Seven hundred fifty-eight million tons of wheat consumption and use are estimated globally in

2020 [12]. Despite this estimation and the importance of wheat in the production of food from an economic, social, technological, and sensory point of view, individuals who have DRGs (celiac disease, non-celiac gluten sensitive, gluten ataxia, wheat allergy, among others) need to exclude these products from their diet [13–15]. Currently, the only treatment for DRGs is the gluten-free diet (GFD) [14, 16]. About 10% of the population adopts a GFD for the treatment of GRD or by option [16, 17]. The complete dietary exclusion of gluten can promote remission of the symptoms. Also, it enables regularization of serological parameters (in case of celiac disease and wheat/gluten allergy), and minimization of the negative repercussions of GRD [18, 19].

The tolerable limit of daily gluten intake by celiacs varies between individuals. The evidence currently available does not yet allow the establishment of an absolute and universal safe value. In a systematic review, it is suggested that some individuals have a good tolerance to 34-36 mg of gluten per day. In comparison, others reveal abnormalities in the intestinal mucosa as a result of consuming only 10 mg of gluten/day [20]. These data show the importance of evaluating and monitoring gluten-free products to guarantee safeness to GRD patients.

According to the Codex Alimentarius Commission [21], 'gluten-free foods' are produced from one or more ingredients that do not contain wheat, rye, barley, and oats or their crossed varieties, and in which the gluten level can not be higher than 20 mg/kg (ppm) in total, based on the portion of the food. 'Gluten-free foods' are also those made with one or more ingredients that contain wheat, rye, barley, and oats or their crossed varieties, which have undergone proper gluten removal, provided that the gluten levels do not exceed 20 mg/kg in total [21].

Adherence to a gluten-free diet, consisting of foods that meet the permitted limit of gluten in foods, is associated with the improvement of physical and physiological aspects of individuals with GRD [22, 23]. Although the treatment for the disease consists of dietary restriction, studies show that by completely excluding gluten from the diet and, consequently, reducing symptoms, many patients can achieve physical and emotional well-being [23–25].

Although GFD is the only treatment for GRD, maintaining a completely gluten-free diet is extremely difficult. Despite the increased availability of food products and gluten-free meals in food services and markets around the world, these gluten-free foods tend to have high cost and compromised nutritional, sensory and technological qualities [1, 26–28].

The supply of products and the emergence of food services for GRD have been growing in recent years, increasing the variety of gluten-free preparations and also improving their sensory aspects [29, 30]. However, it is essential to highlight that the food industry tends to increase the amounts of fats and sugars to mimic the technological characteristics of gluten in the product [31–33].

Despite the increase in gluten-free products on the market, maintaining a DSG still presents challenges, mainly concerning meals in which gluten-containing products are traditional, like breakfast.

BREAKFAST AND GLUTEN-CONTAINING PRODUCTS

Breakfast is described as one of the most important meals of the day, generally consumed before going to work and reaching close to 20% of the nutritional recommendations [34]. Adequate consumption of breakfast also seems to assist in weight control; compared to other daily meals, the morning meal provides a higher intake of vitamins and minerals and a lower intake of fats and cholesterol [35, 36]. Although breakfast is considered one of the main meals of the day, there is a relative lack of information in their gluten-containing products and gluten-free options.

Besides dairy products and fruits, gluten-containing products figure as the most consumed products for breakfast [34, 37, 38]. Bread, cakes, pancakes, cookies, crackers, cereals, toasts, waffles, and others are examples of widely consumed products in breakfast [38]. To the best of our knowledge, there is no scientific study about gluten-free waffles. Therefore, we will discuss other gluten-free breakfast products.

Bread

Bread is a dough based on wheat flour and water, fermented or not, kneaded, and baked [39]. Among the foods known to humanity, bread has been present since the beginning of recorded history, in rites, religious cults, portrayed in fables, and base for the food of different people of different ethnicities [40]. In Europe, the average per capita consumption of bread is 59.4 kg per year [41]. In the United States, consumption reaches up to 25kg per capita in a year, and 179 million Americans usually consume at least one package of bread within a week [42]. In Brazil, bread consumption is also high, reaching 19.3 kg of bread per year [43]. Bread is not only consumed at breakfast, but this meal is the main one for this product's intake in many countries.

In bakery products, gluten performs functions related to stability, growth, texture, toughness, and elasticity, and its presence is essential to obtain these characteristics [44]. In the cooking process of baking doughs, gases are produced from the fermentation and/or steam from the liquids added to the batter. The cohesive and elastic network formed by the gluten expands, retaining these gases in the dough favoring growth [45, 46]. At the same time, due to the heat of the cooking process, coagulation and denaturation of this protein network occurs, favoring that the size obtained during the gas expansion remains at the end of the cooking process, thus resulting in the final growth of the dough [46].

In wheat, a gluten-cereal whose use is more expressive in breadmaking, the gliadin (prolamine) is responsible for the cohesion characteristic of the structure and becomes gummy, dense, and little expandable when hydrated. In contrast, glutenin, formed by numerous chains linked between itself, becomes elastic and accounts for the protein's extensibility [44, 46]. Different wheat flours have different levels of gluten, which vary between 7 to 12%. The higher the gluten content of the flour, the greater the strength of the protein network formed [47]. Thus, wheat flours with lower gluten content are indicated for preparations with a softer final texture (spongy bread, cakes, pancakes, cookies, waffles) and, with higher gluten content, for foods that require more resistance and toughness (some types of bread) [47].

Aiming to meet the need of gluten exclusion of bread and the desire of people who suffer from GRD, researchers and the food industry are searching for a GFB with similar quality aspects of traditional gluten-containing bread [48, 49]. However, most of these products present poor nutritional quality (highly starchy and fatty, and deficient in protein, fiber, and micronutrients) to compensate for the lack of gluten and achieving good acceptance by consumers [50].

Different starch/flour combinations or enrichment agents are used in the formulation of GFB [48, 51, 52] to substitute gluten's technological and sensory characteristics. Rice, potato, corn, and cassava starches are common substitutes in GFB, usually combined in different proportions among them. Their different rheological characteristics (mainly gelatinization and gelation proprieties) contribute to GFB with satisfactory technological and sensory aspects [51, 53, 54]. However, it is essential to highlight that these ingredients present high Glycemic-index (GI) due to their starch content, and the GFB also tend to show high GI [52].

GFB formulations also present protein and fiber. However, high amounts of them can impact on the sensory quality and acceptance of the GFB. Pseudocereals are also used in GFB formulations to improve nutritional quality and the protein structure. However, given their incapacity to form stable structures to produce good quality bread, they are combined with starch sources with enhanced capacity to retain water and form gels [55–59].

A study [60] used the combination of rice and potato starches with different percentages of inulin-type fructan (ITF) to improve the nutritional quality due to its complex carbohydrate chains. ITF is known to act similarly as dietary fiber slowing the process of digestion and absorption of carbohydrates, lowering the GI, promoting gut function regulation, among others [60–62]. Despite the implementation of ITF reducing GI, and potentially improving other physiological functions, higher amounts of IFT impaired sensorial characteristics [60].

The IFT was also used in combination with rice, soy flours, and cassava starch in bread [63], acting as a prophylactic measure to prevent constipation, a common symptom in GRD bearers [64, 65]. Also, its prebiotic potential has proven to enhance the absorption of minerals and to stimulate the immune system [64, 65].

Potato and rice starches were used in combination with different hydrocolloids. Segura et al. [58] analyzed GFB brands available in Spain's local markets. Xanthan and guar gums, carboxymethyl-cellulose (CMC), pectin, and hydroxypropyl-methyl-cellulose (HPMC) were used as gluten replacements and stabilizing agents [56, 58, 66]. They also retarded the releasement of digested carbohydrates since they can form denser, slowly digestible molecules in the presence of protein (like casein milk protein) present in GFB [58]. There is a study evaluating the *Colocasia esculenta* in GFB combined with HPMC, xanthan, and guar gums. However, *Colocasia esculenta* GFB showed compact structures, an undesirable sensory characteristic for bread [66].

Rice flours produced from different cultivars were used as a single starch source in GFB making. Tarom, Hashemi, Khouzestan, and Lenian are Iranian rice cultivars that differ in their nutritional composition since their harvests occur in places with contrasting climates. The first two occur in mild and humid regions, and the last ones grow in dry areas [67]. The GFB made with rice from more waterless places presented higher values of protein and fibers, nutritional compounds [67, 68]. However, GFB made with arid regions' rice cultivars presented lower technological and sensory quality [67].

GFB made from pseudocereals presented GIs classified as high by Wolter et al. [69]. Different fiber, starch, fat, and protein levels are present in each one of the used flours. Quinoa presented lower levels of protein, starch, and fiber; therefore, its digestion is facilitated, resulting in the highest GI of all analyzed samples, followed by the buckwheat flour based GFB [70]. Teff and sorghum flour naturally present more elevated amounts of fiber, complex starches, and protein; therefore ensuing in slower digestion and decreased GI [68, 70, 71].

Other bread formulation presented oats [63, 70]. However, it is important to note that oat's prolamin fraction, avenin, may trigger reactions in some people with GRD, so its use is not recommended in a gluten-free diet [72]. Studies used psyllium in GFB that presents multiple health benefits, mainly related to complications of the gastrointestinal tract, like diarrhea and constipation. Also, psyllium favored the technological and sensory characteristics in this kind of product [51, 54].

Sourdough is traditionally a yeast replacement based on microorganisms colonies from spontaneous growth [59]. Its implementation in bakery products improves digestibility, bioavailability of different nutrients, and, in the context of GFB, better palatability of the products [40, 73]. A study [74] analyzed the available Italian market sourdough GFB based on rice and millet flours, and rice, corn, and potato starches, and in addition to the good sensory quality, these products showed low GI (52) [74].

Several studies have been searching for the ideal combination of ingredients to GFB. However, we do not have a perfect formulation that puts together nutritional, sensory, and technological quality and scientists are still searching for the best combination of ingredients.

Breakfast-Cereals

Breakfast cereals are products based on cereal grains like corn, oats, wheat, rice. Among them, only oats and wheat contain gluten. However, most of the cereals use a mix of grains, and/or are produced in the same equipment/local with gluten-containing products. In this sense, several breakfast-cereal brands present the gluten-containing claim on their label despite breakfast cereals do not directly depend on gluten characteristics. Therefore, most of them are produced or contaminated with gluten-cereals. These products are important for the population due to their innumerous desirable features, such as practicality, convenience, diversified flavors and shapes, shelf-life, and nutritional composition [75].

Recent studies have been looking for new alternatives to gluten-free breakfast cereals [75–77]. In this sense, a study successfully developed breakfast cereals formulated with broken rice grains, passion fruit peel flour and whey powder (ratio of 87:03:10) under controlled temperature and extrusion. This product was considered well-accepted, high in protein (7.55 g/100g), fiber (6.12 g/100g), and mineral content (1.38 g/100g), also low in lipid content (0.97 g/100g)[75].

Another study used extruded black and red whole rice grains to produce gluten-free breakfast cereals [78]. Despite the lack of nutritional information in the study, the authors showed that pigmented rice varieties could be successfully used in the production of attractive natural colored gluten-gree breakfast cereal balls by extrusion with desirable expansion, texture, and color properties.

A study investigated the quality of gluten-free vermicelli (a product used as a breakfast item in Asia) from pearl millet, incorporating defatted soy flour and hydrocolloids [79]. Vermicelli is an extruded dough into long strands and dried. The authors showed that the addition of guar and karaya gum with carboxy-methylcellulose conducted to the production of gluten-free vermicelli. It also decreased the *in vitro* digestibility of protein and starch. The study showed successful production of gluten-free vermicelli with a good amount of protein, minerals, and fibers, potentially presenting health benefits.

According to Bustamante et al. [80] analyzing the evolution of gluten content in cereal-based gluten-free foodstuffs ($n = 3141$), the breakfast cereals food group presented the highest proportion of gluten-detected samples with 21.5% (73/339) of samples contaminated. It reinforces the need for public policies and regulations to avoid food contamination with gluten to GRD individuals.

Pancakes

Pancakes, traditionally served with sweet toppings or a savory filling and coated in a creamy sauce, are prepared from the batter using wheat flour, milk/water, eggs, oil/butter, and fried on a hot plate [81]. Pancake is a popular wheat-based product consumed in some countries for breakfast that must be reformulated to a gluten-free version to attend the GRD individuals. Some studies were conducted to achieve good formulations to replace wheat in pancakes [81–83]. Akshata et al. [81] aimed to compare the quality characteristics of pancake of wheat and rice flour along with whey protein concentrate. Also, the authors studied the effect of green gram split dehusked flour, xanthan gum, sodium stearoyl-2-lactylate, psyllium on the batter, and sensory characteristics of pancake with rice flour and whey protein concentrate. The study successfully demonstrated the use of rice flour as a primary raw material along with green gram split dehusked flour, whey protein concentrate, and the incorporation of xanthan gum, sodium stearoyl-2-lactylate, psyllium husk for the development of gluten-free and eggless pancake [81].

A study evaluated gluten-free pancakes using different ratios of rice and sweet potato flours, and their rheological, nutritional, and textural properties [82]. The GF pancakes formulations used rice flour combined with sweet potato flour at 10, 20, and 40%. The ingredients used in the formulation were: flour (97.7g), salt (2.0g), sugar (19.7g), baking powder (4.2g), and nonfat dried milk (15.0g), water (108.4g) and Egg Beaters (39.1g). Textural analyses showed that hardness and chewiness increased with time after cooking. However, they decreased with an increase in the amount of sweet potato flour. Cohesiveness decreased with time after cooking, rising with the increased proportion of sweet potato flour. The sweet potato flour (20 - 40%) enhanced the hydration capacity of the rice batter and resulted in increased batter viscosity, similar to the traditional wheat dough. Nutritional properties of the GF pancakes (such as protein content, dietary fiber, total carbohydrate, and total energetic value) were similar to their gluten-containing counterpart. Therefore, the use of rice flour combined with sweet potato flour in pancake formulation seems to be interesting to replace wheat [82].

Another study aimed to compare the characteristics of a gluten-free pancake mix to its counterpart through the sensory aspect [83]. The authors showed the preference for the wheat-containing pancakes than the gluten-free ones. The ingredients were similar except for the type of flour and the addition of xantham gum in the gluten-free pancake. The authors concluded that standardized pancakes were preferred in a blind test, indicating the need for additional research to develop a more acceptable gluten-free pancake [83].

Crackers

Crackers are thin crisp wafers or biscuits usually made of unleavened wheat dough, which contain fat in a considerable amount, up to 30%. They are a popular snack for the group of bakery products, consumed in breakfast and along the day [84]. Crackers can be divided into three main categories based on their differences in ingredients and production methods. Saltines or cream crackers (also called soda crackers) are produced using a wheat sponge and dough system fermented for 16–20 hours. The other ingredients are added to the sponge and ferment for another 3–6 hours before baking. Another category is snack crackers, usually chemically leavened using sodium or ammonium bicarbonate in the presence of a food-grade acid for 30 min to 4 hours. The last one is flavored crackers. They are produced like soda crackers, added flavors (cheese and/or spices) [85].

In crackers, the gluten network needs to be only slightly developed for the dough to be cohesive without being too elastic. However, the absence of structure-forming gluten proteins results in weak resistance of the cracker dough, and the production of high-quality gluten-free cracker represents a significant technological challenge [84]. A study developed a gluten-free cracker snack using 100% of pulse flours (desi chickpea, green lentil, red lentil, pinto bean, navy bean, and yellow pea) and yellow pea fractions (protein, fiber, and starch isolates) [85]. The physical and nutritional characteristics of the cracker were similar to the commercial ones, and they were scored highly in consumer acceptance testing, showing that the pulse flours are an excellent alternative to substitute wheat in crackers.

During the soaking and cooking processes of legumes, some water-soluble proteins, carbohydrates, phenolics, and saponins are leached in the water and may act as emulsifiers and antistaling agents. Therefore, a study investigated the composition of soybean cooking water and its physicochemical, pasting properties, and effect in gluten-free crackers during storage [86]. The soybean cooking resulted in a high loss of material in the cooking water, mainly insoluble fiber. The soybean cooking water exerted emulsifying and foaming abilities, attributed to proteins and saponins. Incorporation of soybean cooking water into a gluten-free cracker prevented hardening upon storage and increased softness and moisture content. Nonetheless, improved texture and mineral content, figuring as a good alternative to produce gluten-free crackers [86].

Refined and wholegrain formulations for gluten-free buckwheat crackers were developed compared with wheat-based crackers [84]. Buckwheat-crackers have higher total phenolic and tocopherol content than wheat-crackers as well as the antioxidant activity. Sensory tests showed that buckwheat-crackers were well accepted. The authors stated that the introduction of buckwheat-crackers in the market would increase the diversity of functional bakery gluten-free products [84].

A study developed an antioxidant gluten-free cracker snack with the inclusion of carob germ and seed peel. The authors showed that these ingredients affected significantly nutritional, physicochemical, sensory, and antioxidant parameters. The germ content ranging from 4 to 14% and seed peel lower than 9% were considered optimal formulation of a protein and fiber-rich gluten-free crackers with high antioxidant activity. However, concentration out of the optimal range of germ/peel harmed the color, texture, and flavor of the gluten-free crackers.

Other Gluten-Free Products

Besides looking for gluten-free alternatives for usually consumed food in breakfast, it is essential to emphasize other products commonly present in breakfast around the world that do not present gluten. They can be more accessible options for GRD patients.

Breakfast around the countries varies according to the available food, the climate, cultural aspects, colonization processes, among other influences that make this type of meal even different inside a country. With all these differences, GRD patients live a variety of situations worldwide, and when traveling abroad. Breakfasts present not only gluten products but also recipes containing eggs, cheese, meats, sausages, corn, rice, and legumes. Fruits and vegetables may be part of breakfast naturally or in juices, dishes, or teas.

Some examples are essential to show the variety that we experience in having breakfasts around the globe. It is interesting to see how different cultures interpret their first meal of the day. In Thailand, fish, pork, and rice are served, while in Japan, pork is replaced by tofu. Besides tofu, India presents lentils, veggie sausages, and roasted potatoes. Germany also has sausages for breakfast but made with pork and other types of meat. Germans also add cheese in their breakfast, as well as Turkish and Colombians. In Turkey, olives, eggs, tomatoes, and cucumbers are also present. Corn is an ingredient that also can be a good substitute for bread and cereals in many countries. Mexico has corn tortillas, and Brazil prepares a couscous with cornflour. Brazilians also include cassava, sweet potatoes, pumpkin, and coconut in their meals.

In Africa, each country contributes to a different breakfast. In Egypt, a dish called Faoul Madamas, is prepared with fava beans, chickpeas, garlic, and lemon. Ghana has a recipe called Waakye made with rice and beans, and Uganda a recipe with green bananas cooked with beef. All these examples encourage GRD people to look for not only gluten-free products similar to the gluten-containing options, but also to different ingredients and cultural dishes that can enrich breakfast.

FINAL CONSIDERATIONS

There has been a food industry and researchers' effort to produce gluten-free products with acceptable nutritional, sensory, and technological qualities to compose meals like breakfast. Most of the products used to replace wheat are starches from cereal or pseudocereal grains, as well as legume flours. Also, hydrocolloids are extensible used to replace gluten. Some formulations in breakfast preparations showed health benefits. However, there is a lack of studies regarding the physiological effect of the gluten-free products' consumption, mainly in the first meal of the day. Despite the effort to produce gluten-free goods, it is evident that the lack of gluten impacts negatively on acceptance and technological characteristics. Also, the combination of ingredients rich in starch and lipid seems to present a negative effect on consumers' health. Therefore, it is essential to stimulate the consumption of a balanced diet with a low amount of unhealthy products to GRD individuals.

REFERENCES

[1] Dessì, M.; Noce, A.; Vergovich, S.; Noce, G.; Daniele, N. Di Safety Food in Celiac Disease Patients: A Systematic Review. *Food Nutr. Sci.* 2013, *04*, 55–74, doi:10.4236/fns.2013.47A008.

[2] Patiño-Rodríguez, O.; Arturo Bello-Pérez, L.; Celeste Flores-Silva, P.; María Sánchez-Rivera, M.; Andrea Romero-Bastida, C. *Physicochemical properties and metabolomic profile of gluten-free spaghetti prepared with unripe plantain flours*. 2018, doi:10.1016/j.lwt.2017.12.025.

[3] Van Der Borght, A.; Goesaert, H.; Veraverbeke, W. S.; Delcour, J. A. Fractionation of wheat and wheat flour into starch and gluten: overview of the main processes and the factors involved. *J. Cereal Sci.* 2005, *41*, 221–237, doi:10.1016/J.JCS.2004.09.008.

[4] Gélinas, P.; McKinnon, C. M.; Mena, M. C.; Méndez, E. Gluten contamination of cereal foods in Canada. *Int. J. Food Sci. Technol.* 2008, *43*, 1245–1252, doi:10.1111/j.1365-2621.2007.01599.x.

[5] Koerner, T. B.; Cléroux, C.; Poirier, C.; Cantin, I.; Alimkulov, A.; Elamparo, H. Gluten contamination in the Canadian commercial oat supply. *Food Addit. Contam. Part A* 2011, *28*, 705–710, doi:10.1080/ 19440049.2011.579626.

[6] Farage, P.; Villas Boas, G.; Gandolfi, L.; Pratesi, R.; Zandonadi, R. P. Is the Consumption of Oats Safe for Celiac Disease Patients? A Review of Literature. *J. Food Nutr. Disord.* 2014, *03*, doi:10.4172/ 2324-9323.1000138.

[7] BRASIL, F. I. Panificação- Os ingredientes enriquecedores. *FIB-Food Ingredients Bras.* 2009, 22–27.
[8] Day, L.; Augustin, M. A.; Batey, I. L.; Wrigley, C. W. Wheat-gluten uses and industry needs. *Trends Food Sci. Technol.* 2006, *17*, 82–90, doi:10.1016/j.tifs.2005.10.003.
[9] Silow, C.; Zannini, E.; Axel, C.; Belz, M. C. E.; Arendt, E. K. Optimization of Fat-Reduced Puff Pastry Using Response Surface Methodology. *Foods* 2017, *6*, 15, doi:10.3390/foods6020015.
[10] Abitrigo/MDIC Estimativa De Moagem De Trigo E Consumo De Farinha - 2005 à 2018. [MDIC Estimated Wheat Milling And Flour Consumption]
[11] *Eat Wheat*; Kansas Wheat; Council, W. F. Eat Wheat.
[12] FAO. *FAO Cereal Supply and Demand Brief.*
[13] Cabrera-Chávez, F.; Granda-Restrepo, D. M.; Arámburo-Gálvez, J. G.; Franco-Aguilar, A.; Magaña-Ordorica, D.; Vergara-Jiménez, M. de J.; Ontiveros, N. Self-Reported Prevalence of Gluten-Related Disorders and Adherence to Gluten-Free Diet in Colombian Adult Population. *Gastroenterol. Res. Pract.* 2016, *2016*, 1–8, doi:10.1155/2016/4704309.
[14] Mulder, C. J. J.; Van Wanrooij, R. L. J.; Bakker, S. F.; Wierdsma, N.; Bouma, G. Gluten-free diet in gluten-related disorders. *Dig. Dis.* 2013, *31*, 57–62, doi:10.1159/000347180.
[15] Catassi, C.; Elli, L.; Bonaz, B.; Bouma, G.; Carroccio, A.; Castillejo, G.; Cellier, C.; Cristofori, F.; de Magistris, L.; Dolinsek, J.; Dieterich, W.; Francavilla, R.; Hadjivassiliou, M.; Holtmeier, W.; Körner, U.; Leffler, D. A.; Lundin, K. E. A.; Mazzarella, G.; Mulder, C. J.; Pellegrini, N.; Rostami, K.; Sanders, D.; Skodje, G. I.; Schuppan, D.; Ullrich, R.; Volta, U.; Williams, M.; Zevallos, V. F.; Zopf, Y.; Fasano, A. Diagnosis of Non-Celiac Gluten Sensitivity (NCGS): The Salerno Experts' Criteria. *Nutrients* 2015, *7*, 4966–77, doi:10.3390/nu7064966.
[16] Sapone, A.; Bai, J. C.; Ciacci, C.; Dolinsek, J.; Green, P. H. R.; Hadjivassiliou, M.; Kaukinen, K.; Rostami, K.; Sanders, D. S.; Schumann, M.; Ullrich, R.; Villalta, D.; Volta, U.; Catassi, C.; Fasano,

A. Spectrum of gluten-related disorders: consensus on new nomenclature and classification. *BMC Med.* 2012, *10*, 13, doi:10.1186/1741-7015-10-13.

[17] Lerner, A. Autoimmunity Reviews New therapeutic strategies for celiac disease. *Autoimmun. Rev.* 2010, *9*, 144–147, doi:10.1016/j.autrev.2009.05.002.

[18] Farage, P. *Construção e avaliação de instrumento de verificação de condições e procedimentos relacionados à produção de alimentos isentos de glúten para indivíduos com doença celíaca*, University of Brasília, 2018. [*Construction and evaluation of an instrument to verify conditions and procedures related to the production of gluten-free foods for individuals with celiac disease*]

[19] Barada, K.; Abu Daya, H.; Rostami, K.; Catassi, C. Celiac Disease in the Developing World. *Gastrointest. Endosc. Clin. N. Am.* 2012, *22*, 773–796, doi:10.1016/j.giec.2012.07.002.

[20] Akobeng, A. K.; Thomas, A. G. Systematic review: tolerable amount of gluten for people with coeliac disease. *Aliment. Pharmacol. Ther.* 2008, *27*, 1044–1052, doi:10.1111/j.1365-2036.2008.03669.x.

[21] Codex Alimentarius. *Standard For Foods For Special Dietary Use For Persons Intolerant To Gluten*; 2008;

[22] Skjerning, H.; Mahony, R. O.; Husby, S.; DunnGalvin, A. Health-related quality of life in children and adolescents with celiac disease: patient-driven data from focus group interviews. *Qual. Life Res.* 2014, *23*, 1883–1894, doi:10.1007/s11136-014-0623-x.

[23] Pratesi, C. B.; Häuser, W.; Uenishi, R. H.; Selleski, N.; Nakano, E. Y.; Gandolfi, L.; Pratesi, R.; Zandonadi, R. P. Quality of life of celiac patients in Brazil: Questionnaire translation, cultural adaptation and validation. *Nutrients* 2018, *10*, 1–12, doi:10.3390/nu10091167.

[24] Marchese, A.; Klersy, C.; Biagi, F.; Balduzzi, D.; Bianchi, P. I.; Trotta, L.; Vattiato, C.; Zilli, A.; Rademacher, J.; Andrealli, A.; Astegiano, M.; Michelini, I.; Häuser, W.; Corazza, G. R. Quality of life in coeliac patients: Italian validation of a coeliac questionnaire. *Eur. J. Intern. Med.* 2013, *24*, 87–91.

[25] Chishty, S.; Singh, N. Impact of nutrition and health counselling on quality of life in celiac children aged 7-12 years as reported by parents. *Nutr. Food Sci.* 2019, *49*, 62–74, doi:10.1108/NFS-01-2018-0019.

[26] Falcomer, A. L.; Araújo, L. S.; Farage, P.; Monteiro, J. S.; Nakano, E. Y.; Zandonadi, R. P. Gluten contamination in food services and industry: A systematic review. *Crit. Rev. Food Sci. Nutr.* 2018, *0*, 1–15, doi:10.1080/10408398.2018.1541864.

[27] Mogul, D.; Nakamura, Y.; Seo, J.; Blauvelt, B.; Bridges, J. F. P. The unknown burden and cost of celiac disease in the U.S. *Expert Rev. Pharmacoeconomics Outcomes Res.* 2017, *17*, 181–188, doi:10.1080/14737167.2017.1314785.

[28] Missbach, B.; Schwingshackl, L.; Billmann, A.; Mystek, A.; Hickelsberger, M.; Bauer, G.; König, J. Gluten-free food database: the nutritional quality and cost of packaged gluten-free foods. *PeerJ* 2015, *3*, 1–18, doi:10.7717/peerj.1337.

[29] Valitutti, F.; Iorfida, D.; Anania, C.; Trovato, C. M.; Montuori, M.; Cucchiara, S.; Catassi, C. Cereal Consumption among Subjects with Celiac Disease: A Snapshot for Nutritional Considerations. *Nutrients* 2017, *9*, doi:10.3390/NU9040396.

[30] Rostami, K.; Bold, J.; Parr, A.; Johnson, M. W. *Nutrients*. MDPI AG August 2017,.

[31] Zandonadi, R. P.; Botelho, R. B. A.; Gandolfi, L.; Ginani, J. S.; Montenegro, F. M.; Pratesi, R. Green Banana Pasta: An Alternative for Gluten-Free Diets. *J. Acad. Nutr. Diet.* 2012, *112*, 1068–1072, doi:10.1016/j.jand.2012.04.002.

[32] Pellegrini, N.; Agostoni, C. Nutritional aspects of gluten-free products. *J. Sci. Food Agric.* 2015, *95*, 2380–2385, doi:10.1002/jsfa.7101.

[33] Jamieson, J. A.; Weir, M.; Gougeon, L. Canadian packaged gluten-free foods are less nutritious than their regular gluten-containing counterparts. *PeerJ* 2018, *2018*, doi:10.7717/peerj.5875.

[34] Trancoso, S. C.; Cavalli, S. B.; Proença, R. P. da C. Café da manhã: caracterização, consumo e importância para a saúde. *Rev. Nutr.* 2010, *23*, 859–869, doi:10.1590/S1415-52732010000500016.

[35] Utter, J.; Scragg, R.; Mhurchu, C. N.; Schaaf, D. At-Home Breakfast Consumption among New Zealand Children: Associations with Body Mass Index and Related Nutrition Behaviors{A figure is presented}. *J. Am. Diet. Assoc.* 2007, *107*, 570–576, doi:10.1016/j.jada. 2007.01.010.

[36] Mekary, R. A.; Giovannucci, E.; Cahill, L.; Willett, W. C.; Van Dam, R. M.; Hu, F. B. Eating patterns and type 2 diabetes risk in older women: Breakfast consumption and eating frequency. *Am. J. Clin. Nutr.* 2013, *98*, 436–443, doi:10.3945/ajcn.112.057521.

[37] de Sousa, J. R.; Botelho, R. B. A.; Akutsu, R. de C. C. A.; Zandonadi, R. P. Nutritional Quality of Breakfast Consumed by the Low-Income Population in Brazil: A Nationwide Cross-Sectional Survey. *Nutrients* 2019, *11*, 1418, doi:10.3390/nu11061418.

[38] Bian, L.; Markman, E. M. Why do we eat cereal but not lamb chops at breakfast? Investigating Americans' beliefs about breakfast foods. *Appetite* 2020, *144*, 104458, doi:10.1016/j.appet.2019.104458.

[39] Montebello, N. de P.; Araújo, W. M. C.; Botelho, R. B. A. *Alquimia Dos Alimentos - Série Alimentos e Bebidas - 3ª Ed. 2014*; Senac, Ed.; Senac, 2014;

[40] Poutanen, K.; Flander, L.; Katina, K. Sourdough and cereal fermentation in a nutritional perspective. *Food Microbiol.* 2009, *26*, 693–699, doi:10.1016/j.fm.2009.07.011.

[41] Eglite, A.; Kunkulberga, D. Foodbalt 2017 Bread Choice and Consumption Trends. 2017, doi:10.22616/foodbalt.2017.005.

[42] Statista Amount of bread consumed in the US. *Stat. Res. Dep.* 2019, *1*, 1.

[43] Brasil, I. B. de G. e E. I. *Pesquisa de Orçamentos Familiares 2008-2009*; Ministério.; 2011; Vol. 39; ISBN 9788524042225. [*2008-2009 Household Budget Survey*]

[44] Alvarez, M. D.; Herranz, B.; Fuentes, R.; Cuesta, F. J.; Canet, W. Replacement of Wheat Flour by Chickpea Flour in Muffin Batter: Effect on Rheological Properties. *J. Food Process Eng.* 2017, *40*, 1–13, doi:10.1111/jfpe.12372.

[45] Alvarez-Jubete, L.; Auty, M.; Arendt, E. K.; Gallagher, E. Baking properties and microstructure of pseudocereal flours in gluten-free bread formulations. *Eur. Food Res. Technol.* 2009, doi:10.1007/s00217-009-1184-z.

[46] Zandonadi, R. P.; Botelho, R. B. A.; Araújo, W. M. C. Psyllium as a Substitute for Gluten in Bread. *J. Am. Diet. Assoc.* 2009, doi:10.1016/j.jada.2009.07.032.

[47] Da Costa, M. D. G.; De Souza, E. L.; Stamford, T. L. M.; Andrade, S. A. C. Qualidade tecnológica de grãos e farinhas de trigo nacionais e importados. *Cienc. e Tecnol. Aliment.* 2008, *28*, 220–225, doi:10.1590/S0101-20612008000100031. [Technological quality of domestic and imported wheat grains and flours. *Cienc. and Tecnol. Food*]

[48] Sanchez, H. D.; Osella, C. A.; Torre, M. A. Optimization of Gluten-Free Bread Prepared from Cornstarch, Rice Flour, and Cassava Starch. *J. Food Sci.* 2002, *67*, 416–419, doi:10.1111/j.1365-2621.2002.tb11420.x.

[49] Berti, C.; Riso, P.; Monti, L. D.; Porrini, M. *In vitro* starch digestibility and *in vivo* glucose response of gluten-free foods and their gluten counterparts. *Eur. J. Nutr.* 2004, *43*, 198–204, doi:10.1007/s00394-004-0459-1.

[50] Johnston, C.; Snyder, D.; Smith, C. Commercially available gluten-free pastas elevate postprandial glycemia in comparison to conventional wheat pasta in healthy adults: a double-blind randomized crossover trial. *Food Funct.* 2017, doi:10.1039/C7FO00099E.

[51] Zandonadi, R. P.; Botelho, R. B. A.; Araújo, W. M. C. Psyllium as a Substitute for Gluten in Bread. *J. Am. Diet. Assoc.* 2009, *109*, 1781–1784, doi:10.1016/j.jada.2009.07.032.

[52] Cross, C. Gluten-free industry is healthy, but is the food? *CMAJ* 2013, *185*, 4555, doi:10.1503/cmaj.109-4555.

[53] Aplevicz, K. S.; Demiate, I. M. Caracterização de amidos de mandioca nativos e modificados e utilização em produtos panificados. *Ciência e Tecnol. Aliment.* 2007, *27*, 478–484, doi:10.1590/S0101-20612007000300009. [Characterization of native and modified

cassava starches and use in bakery products. *Science and Technology. Food.*]

[54] Fratelli, C.; Muniz, D. G.; Santos, F. G.; Capriles, V. D. Modelling the effects of psyllium and water in gluten-free bread: An approach to improve the bread quality and glycemic response. *J. Funct. Foods* 2018, *42*, 339–345, doi:10.1016/j.jff.2018.01.015.

[55] Shumoy, H.; Van Bockstaele, F.; Devecioglu, D.; Raes, K. Effect of sourdough addition and storage time on *in vitro* starch digestibility and estimated glycemic index of tef bread. *Food Chem.* 2018, *264*, 34–40, doi:10.1016/j.foodchem.2018.05.019.

[56] Liu, X.; Mu, T.; Sun, H.; Zhang, M.; Chen, J.; Fauconnier, M. L. Influence of different hydrocolloids on dough thermo-mechanical properties and *in vitro* starch digestibility of gluten-free steamed bread based on potato flour. *Food Chem.* 2018, *239*, 1064–1074, doi:10.1016/j.foodchem.2017.07.047.

[57] Novotni, D.; Čukelj, N.; Smerdel, B.; Bituh, M.; Dujmić, F.; Ćurić, D. Glycemic index and firming kinetics of partially baked frozen gluten-free bread with sourdough. *J. Cereal Sci.* 2012, *55*, 120–125, doi:10.1016/j.jcs.2011.10.008.

[58] Matos Segura, M. E.; Rosell, C. M. Chemical Composition and Starch Digestibility of Different Gluten-free Breads. *Plant Foods Hum. Nutr.* 2011, *66*, 224–230, doi:10.1007/s11130-011-0244-2.

[59] Houben, A.; Höchstötter, A.; Becker, T. Possibilities to increase the quality in gluten-free bread production: An overview. *Eur. Food Res. Technol.* 2012, *235*, 195–208, doi:10.1007/s00217-012-1720-0.

[60] Capriles, V. A. J. Effects of prebiotic inulin-type fructans on structure, quality, sensory acceptance and glycemic response of gluten-free breads Food & Function. *Food Funct.* 2013, *4*, 104–110, doi:10.1039/c2fo10283h.

[61] Giuberti, G.; Fortunati, P.; Gallo, A. Can different types of resistant starch influence the *in vitro* starch digestion of gluten free breads? *J. Cereal Sci.* 2016, *70*, 253–255, doi:10.1016/j.jcs.2016.07.001.

[62] Capriles, V. D.; Arêas, J. A. G. Approaches to reduce the glycemic response of gluten-free products: *in vivo* and *in vitro* studies. *Food Funct.* 2016, *7*, 1266–1272, doi:10.1039/C5FO01264C.

[63] Sciarini, L. S.; Bustos, M. C.; Vignola, M. B.; Paesani, C.; Salinas, C. N.; Pérez, G. T. A study on fibre addition to gluten free bread: its effects on bread quality and *in vitro* digestibility. *J. Food Sci. Technol.* 2017, *54*, 244–252, doi:10.1007/s13197-016-2456-9.

[64] Miremadi, F.; Shah, N. P. Applications of inulin and probiotics in health and nutrition. *Int. Food Res. J.* 2012, *19*, 1337–1350, doi:10.1079/NRR2005100.

[65] Omar, M.; Shehzad, A.; Shakeel, A.; Shoaib, M.; Sharif, H. R.; Raza, H.; Rakha, A.; Ansari, A.; Niazi, S. Inulin: Properties, health benefits and food applications. *Carbohydr. Polym.* 2016, *147*, 444–454, doi:10.1016/j.carbpol.2016.04.020.

[66] Calle, J.; Benavent-Gil, Y.; Rosell, C. M. Development of gluten free breads from Colocasia esculenta flour blended with hydrocolloids and enzymes. *Food Hydrocoll.* 2019, *98*, 105243, doi:10.1016/j.foodhyd.2019.105243.

[67] Feizollahi, E.; Mirmoghtadaie, L.; Mohammadifar, M. A.; Jazaeri, S.; Hadaegh, H.; Nazari, B.; Lalegani, S. Sensory, digestion, and texture quality of commercial gluten-free bread: Impact of broken rice flour type. *J. Texture Stud.* 2018, *49*, 395–403, doi:10.1111/jtxs.12326.

[68] Mann, J.; Cummings, J. H.; Englyst, H. N.; Key, T.; Liu, S.; Riccardi, G.; Summerbell, C.; Uauy, R.; van Dam, R. M.; Venn, B.; Vorster, H. H.; Wiseman, M. FAO/WHO Scientific Update on carbohydrates in human nutrition: Conclusions. *Eur. J. Clin. Nutr.* 2007, *61*, S132–S137, doi:10.1038/sj.ejcn.1602943.

[69] Wolter, A.; Hager, A. S.; Zannini, E.; Arendt, E. K. *In vitro* starch digestibility and predicted glycaemic indexes of buckwheat, oat, quinoa, sorghum, teff and commercial gluten-free bread. *J. Cereal Sci.* 2013, *58*, 431–436, doi:10.1016/j.jcs.2013.09.003.

[70] Wolter, A.; Hager, A. S.; Zannini, E.; Arendt, E. K. *In vitro* starch digestibility and predicted glycaemic indexes of buckwheat, oat,

quinoa, sorghum, teff and commercial gluten-free bread. *J. Cereal Sci.* 2013, *58*, 431–436, doi:10.1016/j.jcs.2013.09.003.
[71] Laleg, K.; Cassan, D.; Barron, C.; Prabhasankar, P.; Micard, V. Structural, culinary, nutritional and anti-nutritional properties of high protein, gluten free, 100% legume pasta. *PLoS One* 2016, *11*, 1–19, doi:10.1371/journal.pone.0160721.
[72] Hüttner, E. K.; Arendt, E. K. Recent advances in gluten-free baking and the current status of oats. *Trends Food Sci. Technol.* 2010, *21*, 303–312, doi:10.1016/j.tifs.2010.03.005.
[73] Katina, K.; Arendt, E.; Liukkonen, K. H.; Autio, K.; Flander, L.; Poutanen, K. Potential of sourdough for healthier cereal products. *Trends Food Sci. Technol.* 2005, *16*, 104–112, doi:10.1016/j.tifs.2004.03.008.
[74] Scazzina, F.; Dall'Asta, M.; Pellegrini, N.; Brighenti, F. Glycaemic index of some commercial gluten-free foods. *Eur. J. Nutr.* 2015, *54*, 1021–1026, doi:10.1007/s00394-014-0783-z.
[75] Alonso dos Santos, P.; Caliari, M.; Soares Soares Júnior, M.; Soares Silva, K.; Fleury Viana, L.; Gonçalves Caixeta Garcia, L.; Siqueira de Lima, M. Use of agricultural by-products in extruded gluten-free breakfast cereals. *Food Chem.* 2019, *297*, 124956, doi:10.1016/j.foodchem.2019.124956.
[76] Colgrave, M. L.; Byrne, K.; Blundell, M.; Howitt, C. A. Identification of barley-specific peptide markers that persist in processed foods and are capable of detecting barley contamination by LC-MS/MS. *J. Proteomics* 2016, *147*, 169–176, doi:10.1016/j.jprot.2016.03.045.
[77] Vatanparast, H.; Islam, N.; Patil, R. P.; Shamloo, A.; Keshavarz, P.; Smith, J.; Chu, L. M.; Whiting, S.; Vatanparast, H.; Islam, N.; Patil, R. P.; Shamloo, A.; Keshavarz, P.; Smith, J.; Chu, L. M.; Whiting, S. Consumption of Ready-to-Eat Cereal in Canada and Its Contribution to Nutrient Intake and Nutrient Density among Canadians. *Nutrients* 2019, *11*, 1009, doi:10.3390/nu11051009.
[78] Meza, S. L. R.; Sinnecker, P.; Schmiele, M.; Massaretto, I. L.; Chang, Y. K.; Marquez, U. M. L. Production of innovative gluten-free breakfast cereals based on red and black rice by extrusion processing

technology. *J. Food Sci. Technol.* 2019, *56*, 4855–4866, doi:10.1007/s13197-019-03951-y.

[79] Hymavathy, T. V.; Spandana, S.; Sowmya, S. Effect of hydrocolloids on cooking quality, protein and starch digestibility of ready-to-cook gluten free extruded product | TV | Agricultural Engineering International: CIGR Journal. *Agric Eng Int CIGR J.* 2014, *16*, 119.

[80] Bustamante, M. Á.; Fernández-Gil, M. P.; Churruca, I.; Miranda, J.; Lasa, A.; Navarro, V.; Simón, E. Evolution of gluten content in cereal-based gluten-free products: An overview from 1998 to 2016. *Nutrients* 2017, *9*, doi:10.3390/nu9010021.

[81] Akshata, B.; Indrani, D.; Prabhasankar, P. Effects of ingredients and certain additives on rheological and sensory characteristics of gluten-free eggless pancake. *J. Food Process. Preserv.* 2019, *43*, doi:10.1111/jfpp.14129.

[82] SHIH, F. F.; Truong, V. D.; Daigle, K. W. Physicochemical Properties of Gluten-Free Pancakes From Rice and Sweet Potato Flours. *J. Food Qual.* 2006, *29*, 97–107, doi:10.1111/j.1745-4557.2005.00059.x.

[83] McCormick, R.; Syler, G. P. Sensory Evaluation by College Students of a Gluten-Free Pancake Mix as Compared to a Standard Pancake Mix. *J. Am. Diet. Assoc.* 2010, *110*, A73, doi:10.1016/j.jada.2010.06.275.

[84] Sedej, I.; Sakač, M.; Mandić, A.; Mišan, A.; Pestorić, M.; Šimurina, O.; Čanadanović-Brunet, J. Quality assessment of gluten-free crackers based on buckwheat flour. *LWT - Food Sci. Technol.* 2011, *44*, 694–699, doi:10.1016/j.lwt.2010.11.010.

[85] Han, J. (Jay); Janz, J. A. M.; Gerlat, M. Development of gluten-free cracker snacks using pulse flours and fractions. *Food Res. Int.* 2010, *43*, 627–633, doi:10.1016/j.foodres.2009.07.015.

[86] Serventi, L.; Wang, S.; Zhu, J.; Liu, S.; Fei, F. Cooking water of yellow soybeans as emulsifier in gluten-free crackers. *Eur. Food Res. Technol.* 2018, *244*, 2141–2148, doi:10.1007/s00217-018-3122-4.

In: Breakfast
Editor: Petr Měchura

ISBN: 978-1-53618-500-3
© 2020 Nova Science Publishers, Inc.

Chapter 4

GLUTEN-FREE BREAKFAST IN BRAZILIAN PUBLIC SCHOOLS: THE MENU ADEQUACY TO THE NATIONAL PROGRAM

Iris Veleci da Silva Santos, Ana Luisa Falcomer, Priscila Farage and Renata Puppin Zandonadi
Department of Nutrition, University of Brasília, Brasília, Distrito Federal/Brazil

ABSTRACT

In Brazil, the right to food was included as a fundamental right in the Federal Constitution. Among the Brazilian initiatives that contribute to guaranteeing the Human Right to Adequate Food (HRAF/*DHAA*) is the National School Food Program (NSFP/*PNAE*). Since 2014, offering special menus for children with food restrictions has become mandatory, as in cases of children with gluten-related disorders (GRD). In Brazilian public schools, GRD individuals commonly report that there are not substitutes for the gluten-containing foods offered. In some cases, the meal offered at school represents the main meal for low-income children living in a situation of food scarcity at home. Moreover, when alternative gluten-free food is provided, itis not safe for the students due to issues such as gluten cross-contamination. Therefore, the visibility of the difficulties faced in the implementation of special menus for children with celiac disease in Brazilian public schools can contribute to making the Human Right to Adequate Food a reality for this group.

Keywords: Brazilian public schools; gluten-related disorders; celiac disease; gluten-free diet

INTRODUCTION

A 'school meal' is defined as a meal provided to children by the school (Oostindjer et al. 2017). School meals traditionally include at least one main meal (breakfast and/or lunch). In developing countries where some households face food insecurity, school meal programs primarily aim to prevent children's hunger and undernutrition (Oostindjer et al. 2017), since these conditions in early childhood are associated with poor cognitive development, behavior problems, and learning performance in later childhood.

In Brazil, the right to food was included as a fundamental right in the Federal Constitution. Among the Brazilian initiatives that contribute to guaranteeing the Human Right to Adequate Food (HRAF/*DHAA*) is the National School Food Program (NSFP/*PNAE*) (Araújo, Santos, and Araújo 2011; General Assembly of the United Nations 1948; Brasil 2010). It reinforces the right of all people to adequate and healthy food, and it determines that the Government becomes the guardian of the right and has the responsibility to implement public policies guaranteeing the dignity of the individual (Angelica and Lonchiati 2019).

Food and nutritional security consist of the right of everyone to regular and permanent access to quality food, on sufficient quantity, without compromising access to other essential needs, based on health-promoting food practices that respect cultural diversity and that are environmental, culturally, economically and socially sustainable (Brasil. 2006).

In Brazilian public schools, the Government funds the school meal. Since 2014, offering special menus for children with food restrictions has become mandatory, as in cases of children with gluten-related disorders (GRD). Gluten related disorders are characterized by the group of diseases triggered by gluten, including celiac disease (CD), non-celiac gluten sensitivity (NCGS), gluten ataxia, dermatitis herpetiformis (DH), wheat allergy, among others. Gluten is a protein network (composed by prolamins and glutelins) formed in products that contain cereal grains like wheat, barley, rye, and, in some cases, oats (Farage et al. 2014; Koerner et al. 2011). Although studies are looking for new treatment alternatives for GRDs, the total exclusion of gluten from the diet is still the only safe treatment (Barada et al. 2012; Tonutti and Bizzaro 2014).

In Brazilian public schools, GRD individuals commonly report the absence of substitutes for the gluten-containing foods offered. It is important to mention that, in some cases, the school meal is the main meal consumed on the day among low-income children living in a situation of food scarcity at home. Also, when alternative gluten-free meals are provided, these may not be safe for the students due to the risk of gluten contamination (Falcomer et al. 2018).

Therefore, the visibility of the difficulties faced in the implementation of special menus for children with celiac disease or other GRD in Brazilian public schools can contribute to make the Human Right to Adequate Food a reality for this group. In this sense, this chapter aims to review the history of school meals in Brazil and assess the suitability of gluten-free special menus for public schools' students with gluten-related disorders according to the parameters of the National School Feeding Program in the Brazilian Federal District".

HISTORY OF SCHOOL MEALS IN BRAZIL

In the 1930s to 1940s, food in the public school environment became part of the agenda of social movements, which brought up the topic of school (Peixinho 2013). Schools in a particular way began to organize themselves by setting up "school fund", which aimed to raise money in order to offer food to students. The school fund was maintained by voluntary contributions from local companies and students in a position to contribute. This service provided food to all students, or the neediest, being conditioned to the need and/or availability of resources (Tadahiro Shima 2003). Regarding State participation, the proposal did not materialize, as the Government had no financial resources to these initiatives, despite it recognized the importance of school meals on the permanence of students in schools and the reduction of child malnutrition in the country (DIAS and ESCOUTO 2016).

In 1950, the distribution of school lunches began with the Federal Government supporting the States (Tadahiro Shima 2003). In the Brazilian Northeast region, where food was scarce, a group of children with a higher rate of malnutrition started receiving food during class time. At this moment, the food provided was limited to some industrialized products (wheat flour, powdered milk, and soy) donated by international organizations. Thus, the Federal Government did not buy food but distributed it (DIAS and ESCOUTO 2016).

On March 31, 1955, the Brazilian Government officialized the School Lunch Campaign, under the responsibility of the National Food Commission (CNA), through Legislation No. 37106 (Brasil 1955) being the oldest food supplementation program in the country gained national coverage (Tadahiro Shima 2003)

In the 70's, there was a reduction in international donations, and the Federal Government started to buy Brazilian products for school meals. Despite that, the acquisition of industrialized products represented about 54% of the total expenses with school meals compared to local products. The main products purchased in this period were: peanut candy (paçoca); milk powder; industrialized soup (bean soup with noodles, corn cream soup with soy protein, and cereal with vegetables), cookies, among others (DIAS and ESCOUTO 2016), most of them containing gluten.

Over the years, several denominations were attributed to the operationalization of food in the school environment and, in 1979, what was commonly known as "school lunch", became the National School Food Program officially (Peixinho 2013).

In the 1980s, financial and management decentralization of the National School Food Program (PNAE) was started. The participation of states and municipalities in the actions started, as well as the insertion of social participation in inspection, through the School Food Councils (CAE). Since then, PNAE was committed to respecting the food culture of each Brazilian region and to seeking improvements in the acceptance of meals by the students (Verônica et al. 2013)

With Law 11,947 (July 16, 2009), there was a major advance in the PNAE, which set that 30% of the acquisition of foodstuffs should come from local producers. This new proposal contributed to the achievement of healthy and adequate food in the school environment, using varied foods and respecting healthy cultures, traditions, environment, and habits (Brasil 2009).

This program is managed by the National Education Development Fund of the Ministry of Education (FNDE/MEC), serving students in basic education (kindergarten, elementary school, high school, and youth and adult education) in public and philanthropic schools, through the transfer of financial resources (Brasil 2009). The transfer is made directly to the states and municipalities, based on the School Census carried out in the year before the service. The program is monitored and supervised directly by society, through the School Meals Councils (CAE) and by the FNDE (FNDE 2009).

The PNAE receives a name related to its execution at the state level in each Federated Unit. In the Federal District, the PNAE is called the School Feeding Program of the Federal District (PAE/DF), regulated through Legislation No. 167 (September 10, 2010), which establishes the School Food Manual of the Federal District (SEEGDF 2010).

The PAE/DF is guided by the same principals as PNAE, including the use of healthy, varied, adequate safe food, in accordance with the cultural aspects and traditions of the population. The PAE/DF included 'food and nutrition education' in the teaching-learning process (SEEGDF 2010). In this sense, the theme of healthy and adequate food should be addressed across the curriculum, promoting educational actions (Almeida 2006).

Finally, the guidelines established on the PAE/DF advise that the acquisition of foodstuffs must be diversified (covering all food groups), with preference to foods produced and traded locally, by family farming and family entrepreneurs, in order to promote support for sustainability actions (SEEGDF 2010).

School Meals Menu

School meal menus are planned by dietitians, also responsible for the acquisition and use of basic foodstuffs (FNDE 2009). The food purchased must respect the nutritional references, eating habits, culture, and local food tradition, based on the sustainability and agricultural diversification of the region, on healthy and adequate food (Ginani et al. 2020; FNDE 2009).

It is the dietitians' responsibility to develop a meal that meets at least 20% of the daily nutritional needs of primary education students when they attend school part-time. For indigenous students and for part-time students when two meals are offered, a minimum of 30% of the nutritional needs that must be provided. For children enrolled full time at school, meals should cover 70% of their daily nutritional needs (Ministério da Educação 2013).

According to Law 11,914 (Brasil 2009), school meals cover all food offered in the school environment, regardless of its origin. The menu offered must be following the age group and health status of individuals, including those who need specific attention and those who are in social vulnerability.

The menus are key documents in the operationalization of the program. They must be planned based on information about the type of meal, the name of the dish, the ingredients that compose it and its texture, as well as nutritional information as total energetic value (TEV), macronutrients, priority micronutrients (vitamins A and C, magnesium, iron, zinc, and calcium) and fibers (FNDE 2009). The menus must also present the identification (name and register number) and the signature of the dietitian responsible for its planning (Ministério da Educação 2013).

Food security must be contemplated in all stages of the production of school meals. In this sense, the FNDE (FNDE 2009) prohibits the acquisition of foodstuffs like drinks with low nutritional content (soft drinks, artificial soft drinks, and similar), canned food, sausages, sweets, ready-to-eat dishes, or concentrated foods (powdered or dehydrated for reconstitution) with a high amount of sodium (> 500 mg of sodium per 100 g or ml) or saturated fat (> 5.5 g of saturated fat per 100 g, or 2.75 g of saturated fat per 100 ml). Also, The FNDE requires at least three portions of fruits and vegetables per week (200g/student/week) in the meals in order to ensure a healthy and adequate diet (FNDE 2009).

ASSISTANCE TO STUDENTS WITH SPECIAL DIETARY NEEDS

Food, as it is closely linked to human survival, has always been a matter of great concern. The same applies to food in the school environment, especially when food needs differentiation due to some restrictions required by a student's dietary specific condition (Rosa, Pavão, and Marquezan 2019).

Institutions linked to the protection and assistance of people with special dietary needs consider that the experience of dietary restrictions without the right of access to adequate food, based on public policies, is the main factor of social exclusion characterizing a situation of food and nutritional insecurity, aggravated by the social restrictions imposed on people with organic disabilities (Angelica and Lonchiati 2019).

Public policies that aim at food security and its continuous advances draw attention to the problem of the human right to adequate food and people with special dietary needs (Brasil. 2006). Within the scope of sectoral policies with an interface in food assistance and focus on food security, PNAE presents proposals that may represent advances towards the care of these individuals (Ribeiro et al. 2014).

Children with conditions that require special dietary adequacies (diabetes, hypertension, celiac disease, lactose intolerance, phenylketonuria, and others), may not have a visible deficiency but need educational and food inclusion (Rosa, Pavão, and Marquezan 2019). This inclusion modality is essential not only to preserve children's health at school but mainly to enable a complete physical and cognitive development (Ribeiro et al. 2014).

The inclusion of students with dietary restrictions in the school environment is not just about offering special school lunches, as several diseases need adequate and safe ingredients to produce the meal, as is the case of gluten-related disorders (GRD (Benatti 2018). The gluten-free diet goes beyond the care with food intake, and it demands strict conduct of food handlers in the use of gluten-free ingredients solely, the use of exclusive utensils and equipment, and the prevention of cross-contamination (Petruzzelli et al. 2014; Farage et al. 2018). It is in this perspective that inclusion must prevail (FNDE 2017).

Assistance to students with special dietary needs is a spontaneous demand. In all cases, the school principal will receive a medical report to start the process of meeting the student's food needs. A counter reference between the health and education sectors is necessary for the start of student service in the school environment as established by Law n° 12,982/2014, which determines the mandatory plan of special menus for school meals, ratifying and strengthening the guidelines of the National School Food Program, determined by Law 11,947 / 2009 (FNDE 2017).

SPECIAL MENUS IN BRAZILIAN SCHOOLS

The special school menus are prepared by dietitians when demanded by the student's family (through the presentation of the medical report). In some cases, the special menu has a composition similar to the standard menu. In others, it may be necessary to redesign the entire menu and calculate its nutritional value. After approval, the special menus are explained to the food handlers for the preparation of the meal (Angelica and Lonchiati 2019).

At the time of meal preparation, depending on the number of special menus required, it may be necessary to label the meals to avoid exchanges and accidents, such as allergic reactions that can be dangerous, especially when it comes to children. Intake of inappropriate food by people with special dietary needs may directly affect their psychosocial and cognitive development, in addition to their physical health. That is why it is so important to have a differentiated diet for those who need special attention

(Madalena and Dos 2012). Serving food to students with special dietary needs implies in the planning of menus, which are adapted according to technical criteria and recommendations of the Ministry of Health and Guidelines and Consensus published by medical and scientific entities (FNDE 2017).

In addition, the school must have a specific place to prepare special food to avoid cross-contamination, so that it does not compromise food safety. The Resolution RDC No. 26/2015 states that cross-contamination is associated with all stages of the food production chain through poor hygiene practices (Anvisa 2015). Cross-contamination is defined as the presence of any food allergen not intentionally added to the food as a result of growing, producing, handling, processing, preparing, treating, storing, packaging, transporting, or preserving food, or as a result of environmental contamination (Anvisa 2015).

Thus, all food for students who need a special diet must come with their own menu, planned by a dietitian and in compliance with medical guidelines. The preparations must be produced in a safe place, packed in proper packaging, separated from other foods, named and dated so that there is no confusion at the time of meal offer (Angelica and Lonchiati 2019).

Dietary care includes the complete exclusion of allergens in food and the use of exclusive utensils (sponge, cutlery, plastic pots, planks, bottles, blender cups, and mixer). Glass and stainless steel utensils, if well sanitized, can be of common use, but food cannot be prepared together (FNDE 2017).

Another challenge for the school foodservice is the quantitative forecast of the acquisition of differentiated foodstuffs. In general, these foods are not part of the usual school menu but will be necessary for the adaptation of the special menus. They may range from common foods that are not purchased due to high cost, such as olive oil and flaxseed, to specific foods, such as infant formulas or gluten-free products (Angelica and Lonchiati 2019).

Gluten Related Disorders and the Gluten-Free Diet

Celiac disease (CD) is an autoimmune disorder that affects genetically predisposed individuals, caused by permanent intolerance to gluten, the main protein complex fraction present in wheat, rye, barley, oats, and malt (a by-product of barley). The Clinical Protocol and Therapeutic Guidelines (PCDT) was established for the management of CD in Brazil through Ordinance / SAS / MS n° 1149 (BRASIL. MS 2015). In addition to Celiac Disease, there are other gluten-related disorders (GRD), such as non-celiac wheat/gluten sensitivity (NCGS), gluten ataxia, and wheat allergy. Despite immunological differences, all those conditions have a common treatment based on a strict gluten-free diet (Benatti 2018).

Wheat allergy (WA) is a hypersensitivity reaction to wheat protein - gliadins, particularly ѡ 5-Gliadin (the main wheat-dependent allergen). It is a food allergy in which the individual may be sensitized by exposure through the skin or airways (baker's asthma), typical of an IgE-mediated allergy. In WA, symptoms develop within minutes to hours after eating wheat, and they include gastrointestinal, skin and respiratory manifestations, with a risk of death due to anaphylaxis. NCGS may also present with gastrointestinal or extraintestinal manifestations. Since there are no specific markers for it, the diagnosis of NCGS is based on the symptoms described by the patient, when the possibility of CD and WA has been excluded (Guerra 2017).

In WA, wheat exclusion (in some cases, cross-reaction to barley and rye) is necessary, making the diet less restrictive. Unlike CD, this restriction may not be definitive, since the development of tolerance may occur. As to NCGS, the treatment requires a gluten-free diet. However, the rigidity of this food restriction is not yet well defined. It is also unclear so far when the diet needs to be implemented and how to monitor the response to treatment (Guerra 2017).

Although the importance of the gluten-free diet is well established in the literature for the management of GRD, diet compliance rates may vary a lot among patients. A Brazilian study including 34 children and 29 adolescents diagnosed with CD treated consecutively and undergoing treatment for more than 12 months, at the Pediatric Gastroenterology Outpatient Clinic of Escola Paulista de Medicina (Unifesp), showed that a total of 41.2% (n=14) of children and 34.5% (n=10) of adolescents transgressed the gluten-free diet (Andreoli et al. 2013).

Low gluten-free diet adherence may be related to the social and emotional burden that the food restriction generates. A Canadian study conducted with members of two Canadian celiac associations assessed the emotional impact of the difficulties experienced in daily food-related situations by Canadians with celiac disease who followed a gluten-free diet. Among the reported difficulties, the authors found: limited food options in foodservice (87.5%); limited restaurant choices (76.9%); being concerned that gluten does not always appear on food labels (78.9%); high cost of gluten-free foods (61.1%); not liking others feeling sorry for them; worrying about staff in restaurants not being trained in preparing gluten-free meals (63.7%); limited choices in the school/work cafeteria (84.8%); not being able to eat many local/national special dishes (61%), and having to bring their own food to school/work (33.5%) (Zarkadas et al. 2013).

Foods commonly used as substitutes for primary foods that contain gluten (wheat, oats, rye, barley, and malt) are rice (grain, flour, powdered brown rice); corn (flour, flakes, cornmeal, starch, hominy, popcorn); cassava (flour, starch, sweet and sour starch, arrowroot, tapioca); potato starch; millet; quinoa; amaranth; buckwheat; and mixtures of them. Many foodstuffs are naturally gluten-free and can be used to prepare gluten-free dishes, as long as the packaging displayed the inscription "does not contain gluten"/"gluten-free" and there are no traces of wheat, oats, barley or rye (Benatti 2018).

It is also important that the handling of gluten-free food is done with tools for exclusive use. These include skimmers, filters, plates, pots, pans, meat and vegetable chopping boards, pots with lids, tongs, among others. When preparing a gluten-free meal, food handling must be carried out following an orderly and sequential process flow to avoid cross-contamination. The written recipes must be updated and available for consultation by the handler responsible for preparing gluten-free meals. It is necessary to include all process steps to prepare the dish, pointing out the most critical points to avoid cross-contamination (Brasil 2012).

EVALUATION OF BREAKFAST GLUTEN-FREE SPECIAL MENUS IN PUBLIC SCHOOLS FROM THE FEDERAL DISTRICT OF BRAZIL

In the Federal District of Brazil, where the national capital is located, the PNAE is contemplated by the PAE/DF. In order to implement the human right to food access and the program's agenda, a team of dietitians plans the school meal menus considering the population nutritional needs, and also its eating habits, culture, and tradition, and taking into account sustainability issues (FNDE 2009; Ginani et al. 2020).

As previously mentioned, the school menus must contribute to the daily nutritional needs of the students enrolled. For that purpose, children receive one to two meals per day in school. The frequency and the overall percentage of nutrients daily granted vary according to the ethnic population, age, and time spent in school (part-time or full time) (Ministério da Educação 2013).

Brazilian food guideline considers healthy eating as one of the determinants of good health. It also emphasizes that breakfast is one of the three most important meals of the day and suggests meals according to Brazilians food habits (Brasil 2014). Even though the national guideline underlines the importance of breakfast, the PNAE does not have a specific recommendation for this meal (FNDE 2009).

Considering children's need for nutritionally balanced food, it is important to highlight that kids with special dietary needs require food adaptations in order to obtain adequate healthy meals. In regards to children with GRD, aspects such as susceptibility to malnutrition due to small bowel mucosal damage, inability to access gluten-free products due to its higher cost, and restricted food options must be considered for the elaboration of a well-designed meal plan.

For those reasons, the evaluation of school breakfast menus' quality and adapted special menus for kids with GRD is fundamental. Therefore, analysis of the gluten-free breakfast provided in the public schools of the Federal District of Brazil was carried out. For this purpose, all original and gluten-free adapted menus outlined by the PAE/DF and implemented in all the 14 regions of the Federal District during the 11 months of school from February to December (2019) were considered.

The meals offered as breakfast in the schools were composed of a main dish and a complement (beverage). Data analysis show that in the original menus, biscuits (most of them gluten-containing) were present in 85.04% (n=273) of the meals provided, varying between four types of biscuits: 36.26% of sweet buttery biscuits (n=99); 15.02% of corn starch and wheat flour-based biscuits (*biscoito de maisena*) (n=41), 26.74% of salty crackers (*biscoito cream cracker*) (n=73), and 21.98% corn starch based biscuits (*sequilhos*) (n=60). A total of 14.96% (n=48) of breakfast menus include gluten-containing bread, which is offered in two versions, bread accompanied by a protein option (81.25%, n=39) and bread with vegetable pate (18.75%, n=9).

The beverage options vary between coffee with milk, juices, smoothies, and caramelized milk. Juices and smoothies are prepared with fresh fruits and added sugar, without specification of the amount of sugar.

In cases of students with GRD, the meals are adjusted to the following dishes: corn starch-based biscuits (8.06%, n=5), cassava starch biscuits (16.14%, n=10), *cuscuz* (prepared with cornflour) (12.9%, n=8), rice pasta (38,7%, n=24), soup with rice pasta (3.23%, n=2) or tapioca served with a protein option or butter (20.97%, n=13).

It is noticeable that gluten-free food alternatives in school menus are mainly composed of simple carbohydrates and tend to have more fat in order to obtain similar texture as of gluten-containing preparations (Missbach et al. 2015). As a consequence, meals may become abundant in non-nutritional calories. Furthermore, it may not present critical nutrients such as proteins which are so important for children, especially for those who are part of the sociable vulnerable population (Missbach et al. 2015; Oostindjer et al. 2017).

Taking into account that celiacs are part of the group with GRD, it is primordial to consider the group's physiological characteristics. Since CD is an intestinal pathology that causes mucosal damage and is associated with malnutrition due to the inability to absorb nutrients, offering nutritionally adequate food is essential to ensure the health and avoid the consequences of malnutrition such as iron and calcium deficiencies (Sapone et al. 2012).

As a consequence of mucosal damage, celiacs may present lactose intolerance and, therefore, require lactose and gluten-free diet (Collin et al. 2015). However, when a child presents both restrictions, the school meal is adapted to either a fruit or juice. These options are not sources of calcium and protein, thus they are not an adequate substitute to milk preparations. In addition, as the juices may be made from powdered juice mixes, it might not have any nutritional value at all.

For those reasons, special school menus for GRD in Brazil require some adjustments. The last edition of the Brazilian Nutritional Guide (Brasil 2014) presents suggestions to a balanced breakfast and takes into consideration the population food culture and habits. According to the guide, bread is usually substituted by *cuscuz* (prepared with corn flour), *tapioca* (prepared with cassava starch), or cheese bread (prepared with cassava starch), which are all naturally gluten-free options (Brasil 2014). Then, it is viable to apply those national food habits to school meal menus, replacing the most frequent food that is wheat bread by the three mentioned options that are all made of non-expensive ingredients.

Besides the adequacy of the gluten substitutes to the national habits, changes of gluten-containing food in the regular school menus to natural gluten-free options for all the students may help children with special dietary needs feel more included, reducing the feeling of being different and even bullying due to having an unusual diet (Skjerning et al. 2014). Nonetheless, improving the gluten-free options to more nutritional ones and also establishing natural gluten-free options in the original menus may contribute to GRD children's overall health and cognitive development, while possibly minimizing the risk for gluten cross-contamination due to simultaneous preparation of gluten-free and gluten-containing meals in the school canteens.

REFERENCES

Almeida, Gisella de Souza. 2006. "Uma Escola Inclusiva de Referência No Contexto Da Educação Especial No Estado de Goiás: Um Estudo de Caso." *Dados*. ["An Inclusive Reference School in the Context of Special Education in the State of Goiás: A Case Study." *Dice.*]

Andreoli, Cristiana Santos, Ana Paula Bidutte Cortez, Vera Lucia Sdepanian, and Mauro Batista De Morais. 2013. "Avaliação Nutricional e Consumo Alimentar de Pacientes Com Doença Cel Íaca Come Sem Transgressão Alimentar." *Revista de Nutricao* 26 (3): 301–11. https://doi.org/10.1590/S1415-52732013000300005. [Nutritional Assessment and Food Consumption of Patients With Celiac Disease Eats Without Food Transgression. *Journal of Nutrition*]

Angelica, Fabrizia, and Bonatto Lonchiati. 2019. "A Inclusão Alimentar De Alérgicos No Ambiente Escolar." *Revista Jurídica Da UniFil Revista Ju*: 59–94. https://doi.org/ISSN 2674-7251. [The Food Inclusion of Allergies in the School Environment. *Legal Journal Of UniFil Magazine*]

Anvisa. 2015. *Resolução - Rdc Nº 26, De 2 De Julho De 2015 - Anvisa*, 26–29. [*Resolution - Rdc No. 26, of July 2, 2015 – Anvisa*]

Araújo, F. R., D. F. Santos, and M. A. D. Araújo. 2011. "O Direito Humano à Alimentação Adequada Promovido Por Políticas de Acesso a Alimentos: O Caso Da Unidade Natal-RN Do Projeto Café Do Trabalhador." *Revista de Políticas Públicas* 15 (2): 267–76. ["The Human Right to Adequate Food Promoted by Access to Food Policies: The Case of the Natal-RN Unit of the Coffee Worker Project." *Public Policy Review*]

Barada, Kassem, Hussein Abu Daya, Kamran Rostami, and Carlo Catassi. 2012. "Celiac Disease in the Developing World." *Gastrointest Endoscopy Clin N Am* 22: 773–96. https://doi.org/10.1016/j.giec.2012.07.002.

Benatti, Raquel Candido Benati Ester Candido. 2018. *Atendimento Dos Alunos Celíacos No Programa*. www.Riosemgluten.Com.Br. [*Service of Celiac Students in the Program.*]

Brasil. 2006. "Lei Orgânica de Segurança Alimentar e Nutricional. Lei N° 11.346." *Lei Orgânica de Segurança Alimentar e Nutricional. Lei N° 11.346 de 15 de Setembro de 2006. Cria o Sistema Nacional de Segurança Alimentar e Nutricional – SISAN Com Vistas Em Assegurar o Direito Humano à Alimentação Adequada e Dá Outras Providências*, 28. https://doi.org/10.1007/978-3-642-37117-2_17. ["Organic Law on Food and Nutritional Security. Law No. 11,346." *Organic Law on Food and Nutritional Security. Law No. 11,346 of September 15, 2006. Creates the National System of Food and Nutritional Security - SISAN With Views in Ensuring the Human Right to Adequate Food and Provides Other Provisions*]

BRASIL. MS. 2015. *Protocolo Clínico e Diretrizes Terapêuticas Doença Celíaca Portaria SAS/MS N° 1149, de 11 de Novembro de 2015. Revoga a Portaria N° 307/SAS/MS, de 17 de Setembro de 2009. 1.* [*Clinical Protocol and Therapeutic Guidelines Celiac Disease Ordinance SAS / MS No. 1149, of 11 November 2015. Revokes Ordinance No. 307 / SAS / MS, of 17 September 2009. 1.*]

Brasil. 1955. "Decreto N° 37.106, de 31 de Março de 1955." *Diário Oficial Da União*, no. Seção 1-2/4/1955: 0. [Decree No 37.106, of March 31, 1955. *Official Gazette of the Union*, no. Section 1-2 / 4/1955: 0.]

———. 2009. "Lei N° 11.947/2009 – PNAE." *Pnae*, 1–8.

———. 2010. *Decreto N° 7234, de 19 de Julho de 2010. PNAE*. Presidência da República. [*Decree No 7234, of 19 July 2010. PNAE.*]

———. 2012. *Manual de Orientação Sobre Alimentação Escolar Para Portadores de Diabetes, Hipertensão, Doença Celíaca, Fenilcetonúria e Intolerância a Lactose*. Ministério Da Saúde, Secretaria de Atenção à Saúde, Departamento de Atenção Básica, 54. [*School Feeding Guidance Manual for People with Diabetes, Hypertension, Celiac Disease, Phenylketonuria and Lactose Intolerance. Ministry of Health, Department of Health Care, Department of Primary Care*]

———. 2014. *Guia Alimentar Para a População Brasileira Guia Alimentar Para a População Brasileira*. Ministério Da Saúde, Secretaria de Atenção à Saúde, Departamento de Atenção Básica. Vol. 2. [*Food Guide for the Brazilian Population Food Guide for the Brazilian Population.*

Ministry of Health, Department of Health Care, Department of Primary Care.]

Collin, Pekka, Katri Kaukinen, Matti Valimaki, and Jorma Salmi. 2015. "Endocrinological Disorders and Celiac Disease." *Endocrine Reviews* 23 (4): 464–83. https://doi.org/10.1210/er.2001-0035.

DIAS, Barbosa Luciana, and Santos Fernando Luiz ESCOUTO. 2016. "Um Breve Historico Sobre Alimentação Escolar No Brasil." *Faip*, 1–9.

Falcomer, Ana Luísa, Letícia Santos Araújo, Priscila Farage, Jordanna Santos Monteiro, Eduardo Yoshio Nakano, and Renata Puppin Zandonadi. 2018. "Gluten Contamination in Food Services and Industry: A Systematic Review." *Critical Reviews in Food Science and Nutrition*, December, 1–15. https://doi.org/10.1080/10408398.2018.1541864.

Farage, Priscila, Gabriella Villas Bôas, Yanna Karla Nóbrega Medeiros, Riccardo Pratesi, Lenora Gandolfi, and Renata Zandonadi. 2014. *Is the Consumption of Oats Safe for Celiac Disease Patients? A Review of Literature*, 1–9.

Farage, Priscila, Renata Puppin Zandonadi, Verônica Cortez Ginani, Lenora Gandolfi, Eduardo Yoshio Nakano, and Riccardo Pratesi. 2018. "Gluten-Free Diet: From Development to Assessment of a Check-List Designed for the Prevention of Gluten Cross-Contamination in Food Services." *Nutrients* 10 (9). https://doi.org/10.3390/nu10091274.

FNDE. 2009. "Ministério Da Educação Fundo Nacional de Desenvolvimento Da Educação Conselho Deliberativo Resolução/Cd/Fnde N." *Resolução/CD/FNDE Nº38* 38 (1): 1–63. ["Ministry of Education National Fund for the Development of Education Deliberative Council Resolution / Cd / Fnde N." *Resolution / CD / FNDE No 38*]

———. 2017. "Necessidades Alimentares Especiais." *FNDE- Fundo Nacional de Desenvolvimento Da Educação* 1: 64. [Special Food Needs. *FNDE- National Education Development Fund*]

General Assembly of the United Nations. 1948. *Universal Declaration of Human Rights*. Edited by General Assembly of the United Nations. New York.

Ginani, Verônica Cortez, Wilma Maria Coelho Araújo, Renata Puppin Zandonadi, and Raquel B. Assunção Botelho. 2020. "Identifier of Regional Food Presence (IRFP): A New Perspective to Evaluate Sustainable Menus." *Sustainability* 12 (10): 3992. https://doi.org/10.3390/su12103992.

Guerra, et al. 2017. *Doenças Relacionadas Ao Glúten* 27 (Supl 3): 51–58. https://doi.org/10.5935/2238-3182.20170030. [*Gluten-Related Diseases*]

Koerner, T.B., C. Cléroux, C. Poirier, I. Cantin, A. Alimkulov, and H. Elamparo. 2011. "Gluten Contamination in the Canadian Commercial Oat Supply." *Food Additives & Contaminants: Part A* 28 (6): 705–10. https://doi.org/10.1080/19440049.2011.579626.

Madalena, Maria, and Monteiro Dos. 2012. *Um Estudo Sobre a Necessidade De Dietas Especiais Na.* [*A Study on the Need for Special Diets in*]

Ministério da Educação, FNDE. 2013. "Resolução N°26 de 17 de Junho de 2013.Dispõe Sobre o Atendimento Da Alimentação Escolar Aos Alunos Da Educação Básica No Âmbito Do Programa Nacional de Alimentação Escolar – PNAE." *Diário Oficial Da União*, no. D: 1–44. [Resolution N° 26 of June 17, 2013. Provides for the provision of school meals to students of basic education within the scope of the National School Food Program - PNAE. *Official Diary of the Union*]

Missbach, B., L. Schwingshackl, A. Billmann, A. Mystek, M. Hickelsberger, G. Bauer, and J. König. 2015. "Gluten-Free Food Database: The Nutritional Quality and Cost of Packaged Gluten-Free Foods." *PeerJ* 3 (1337): 1–18. https://doi.org/10.7717/peerj.1337.

Oostindjer, Marije, Jessica Aschemann-Witzel, Qing Wang, Silje Elisabeth Skuland, Bjørg Egelandsdal, Gro V. Amdam, Alexander Schjøll, et al. 2017. "Are School Meals a Viable and Sustainable Tool to Improve the Healthiness and Sustainability of Children's Diet and Food Consumption? A Cross-National Comparative Perspective." *Critical Reviews in Food Science and Nutrition* 57 (18): 3942–58. https://doi.org/10.1080/10408398.2016.1197180.

Peixinho, Albaneide Maria Lima. 2013. "A Trajetória Do Programa Nacional de Alimentação Escolar No Período de 2003-2010: Relato Do

Gestor Nacional." *Ciencia e Saude Coletiva* 18 (4): 909–16. ["The Trajectory of the National School Meals Program in the 2003-2010 Period: Report by the National Manager." *Collective Health and Science*]

Petruzzelli, Annalisa, Martina Foglini, Francesca Paolini, Marisa Framboas, M. Serena Altissimi, M. Naceur Haouet, Piermario Mangili, et al. 2014. "Evaluation of the Quality of Foods for Special Diets Produced in a School Catering Facility within a HACCP-Based Approach: A Case Study." *International Journal of Environmental Health Research* 24 (1): 73–81. https://doi.org/10.1080/09603123.2013.782605.

Ribeiro, Cilene Da Silva Gomes, Maria Teresa Gomes de Oliveira Ribas, Carla Corradi-Perini, and Flavia Auler. 2014. "Necessidades Alimentares Especiais Em Ambiente Escolar: Um Ensaio Sobre a Interface Entre Nutrição E Bioética." *DEMETRA: Alimentação, Nutrição & Saúde* 9 (3): 633–44. https://doi.org/10.12957/demetra.2014.10383. ["Special Food Needs in the School Environment: An Essay on the Interface between Nutrition and Bioethics." *DEMETRA: Food, Nutrition & Health*]

Rosa, Mileni da Silveira Fernandes, Sílvia Maria de Oliveira Pavão, and Lorena Ines Peterini Marquezan. 2019. "Alimentação Para Alunos Com Necessidades de Alimentação Especial Como Preceito Educacional Inclusivo." *Revista on Line de Política e Gestão Educacional* 23 (3): 656–64. https://doi.org/10.22633/rpge.v23i3.12573. ["Food for Students with Special Food Needs as an Inclusive Educational Precept." *Online Magazine of Educational Policy and Management*]

Sapone, Anna, Julio C Bai, Carolina Ciacci, Jernej Dolinsek, Peter H R Green, Marios Hadjivassiliou, Katri Kaukinen, et al. 2012. "Spectrum of Gluten-Related Disorders: Consensus on New Nomenclature and Classification." *BMC Medicine* 10 (February): 13. https://doi.org/10.1186/1741-7015-10-13.

SEEGDF, Secretaria de Estado de Educação - Governo do Distrito Federal. 2010. *Manual Da Alimentação Escolar* 55. [State Secretariat of Education - Federal District Government. 2010. *School Feeding Manual*]

Skjerning, Halfdan, Ruth O. Mahony, Steffen Husby, and Audrey DunnGalvin. 2014. "Health-Related Quality of Life in Children and Adolescents with Celiac Disease: Patient-Driven Data from Focus Group Interviews." *Quality of Life Research* 23 (6): 1883–94. https://doi.org/10.1007/s11136-014-0623-x.

Tadahiro Shima, Walter. 2003. *Caminhos Da Alimentação Escolar No Brasil: Análise De Uma Política Pública No Período.* [*Paths of School Feeding in Brazil: Analysis of Public Policy in the Period.*]

Tonutti, Elio, and Nicola Bizzaro. 2014. "Diagnosis and Classification of Celiac Disease and Gluten Sensitivity." *Autoimmunity Reviews* 13 (4–5): 472–76. https://doi.org/10.1016/j.autrev.2014.01.043.

Verônica, Flávia, Marques Calasans, Sandra Maria Chaves, and Dos Santos. 2013. *Avaliação Do Programa Nacional de Alimentação Escolar: Desenvolvimento de Um Protocolo de Indicadores* [*An Evaluation of the National School Meal Program: Development of a Protocol of Indicators*] 20 (1): 24–40.

Zarkadas, M., S. Dubois, K. MacIsaac, I. Cantin, M. Rashid, K. C. Roberts, S. La Vieille, S. Godefroy, and O. M. Pulido. 2013. "Living with Coeliac Disease and a Gluten-Free Diet: A Canadian Perspective." *Journal of Human Nutrition and Dietetics* 26 (1): 10–23. https://doi.org/10.1111/j.1365-277X.2012.01288.x.

In: Breakfast
Editor: Petr Měchura

ISBN: 978-1-53618-500-3
© 2020 Nova Science Publishers, Inc.

Chapter 5

DAIRY PRODUCTS IN BREAKFAST AND THEIR SUBSTITUTES IN THE MILK RESTRICTION DIET

Priscila Farage[1], Luana Rincon[2], Renata Puppin Zandonadi[2], and Raquel Braz Assunção Botelho[2],*

[1]Federal University of Goiás, Goiânia, GO, Brazil
[2]University of Brasília, Brasília, DF, Brazil

ABSTRACT

Breakfast is considered the most important meal of the day. Breakfast options vary a lot worldwide according to cultural feeding habits in different populations. However, milk and its derived products are a common food choice across countries. Milk as a drink is usually consumed with coffee or pure, or it might be combined with cereals in a bowl. Other alternatives include milk derivatives such as yogurt and curd, which may be ingested pure, served with fruits and bread, and used to prepare

* Corresponding Author's E-mail: raquelbabotelho@gmail.com

smoothies. Different types of cheese are also commonly present in the population breakfast. Additionally, there are many other food options, which include milk or other milk ingredients in their recipes. The cultural presence of milk in the diet and its extensive use in the food industry, in general, make it complicated for people who need to adopt a milk-free diet. Some conditions, such as cow's milk allergy and lactose intolerance, demand a restriction of milk in the diet. Vegetarian individuals also restrict milk as a lifestyle choice. In these cases, non-dairy derived substitute products may appear in the individual's diet. However, cow's milk and its derivatives display sensorial features appreciated by the population and essential nutritional characteristics, such as its high protein and calcium content. Therefore, it is important to find viable options with sensory and nutritional quality that can be part of the diet of individuals who restrict milk.

Keywords: breakfast, milk-free diet, plant-based milk, dairy-free products, cow's milk allergy, lactose intolerance

BREAKFAST FOOD AND NUTRIENTS CHARACTERISTICS

Breakfast, as the first meal of the day, is responsible for providing 20–25% of total daily energy through the ingestion of cereals, fruit, and dairy products [1]. Eating breakfast is considered a predictor of healthy eating behavior [2]. This vital meal provides essential nutrients to support adequate growth and energy refuel after long hours of sleep [3].

Individuals who consume breakfast are more likely to have higher intakes of micronutrients and a lower intake of fat, and they also present higher chances of having a better overall diet quality [4]. Skipping breakfast has been associated with weight gain, increased body mass index, higher prevalence of obesity, hypertension, hyperlipidemia, insulin insensitivity, type 2 diabetes, and cardiovascular disease [2].

In the study by Matthys et al. (2007), Belgian adolescents participated in a 7-day estimated food record to obtain a description of their breakfast consumption patterns on a nutrient and food item level. The authors observed that a good-quality breakfast rich in cereals, dairy products, and fruits/vegetables resulted in higher intakes of protein, iron, calcium, magnesium, vitamin B1, vitamin B2, and vitamin C [4].

In children and adolescents, the consumption of breakfast is especially crucial due to physical and mental development processes undergoing these periods of life. Diet and eating practices that are established during these years are likely to persist throughout life [2]. Moreover, eating breakfast has been positively associated with improved cognitive and academic performance, psychosocial function, and school attendance [4].

Although breakfast is important for delivering essential nutrients and energy, it should be mentioned that its nutrient profile may vary according to cultural food habits worldwide and to the stage of life, among other interfering factors. In the study by Al-Hazzaa et al. (2020), the authors investigated breakfast consumption patterns among Saudi primary-school children. The authors pointed out the concerning proportion of children who skipped daily breakfast (79%), which might implicate in children's school performance. Data also showed that spread cheese sandwiches were consumed most frequently among breakfast eaters, followed by fried egg sandwiches and breakfast cereals. The most consumed drinks were full-fat milk, tea with milk, water, and fruit juice [3].

In a cross-sectional survey conducted by Champilomati et al. (2020) including 1,728 Greek children aged 10–12 years, the type of identified breakfast foods included milk (77.8%) or chocolate milk (15.1%) (full fat or light), yogurt (9.9%), cereals (67.7%), fruit juice (27.2%), honey/jam (30.4%), bread/rusks (28.7%), butter/margarine (11.0%) and various types of cake/bagel or tsoureki (21.8%) (a type of sweet brioche) [5].

In France, a nationally representative cross-sectional survey showed that the vast majority of participants were regular consumers of breakfast (5–7 times per week). Data from the 7-day dietary record used in the study to evaluate children, adolescents, and adults' breakfast consumption revealed that breakfast contributed with higher proportions in the daily intake of B and C vitamins, and minerals (calcium, iron, iodine, manganese, phosphorus, potassium, magnesium). The better quality of the diet was associated with higher intakes of whole-grain products (bread and cereals), dairy (milk, fresh dairy), and fruit at breakfast. Milk was responsible for

61.7% of the calcium intake for the group of children and adolescents. Among adults, milk contributed to 41.2% of the calcium ingestion [6].

In Chile, breakfast dietary patterns and their nutritional quality were evaluated among Chilean university students aged 18-27 years old using a breakfast food survey. Data showed that 53% of participants ate breakfast daily; 68% did not consume fruits, and only 17.5% had good breakfast quality. Dairy products and ham were the primary protein sources in this meal. In general, breakfast quality was found inadequate due to low fruit consumption and energy intake. All dietary patterns identified included cereals, bread, dairy, fats, and sugars. Such investigations may be useful for planning future interventions targeted at the improvement of breakfast quality [7].

Ramos et al. [8] evaluated breakfast consumption in the Brazilian low-income population and dairy products were mainly consumed by 54.3% o males and 61.9% of females. Consumption of dairy products increases with age, reaching 68.3% of consumption in participants over 65 years, and with income. Cereals are the second consumed group (male-56.5%; female-58.3%), followed by fruits (male- 18.1%; female – 16.9%).

Ruiz et al. (2018) investigated energy, nutrient, and food group intakes at breakfast in Spain, and the relationship to the overall diet quality (9–75 years old individuals). The majority of the Spanish population (>85%) were regular breakfast consumers. Chocolate (mainly as chocolate-flavored milk and powder) was the most commonly consumed breakfast food among children and adolescents, followed by bakery and pastry, whole milk, and semi-skimmed milk. In older individuals, a wider variety of food options was identified, including bakery and pastry, white bread, semi-skimmed milk, whole milk, butter/margarine, olive oil, and chocolates. An important finding was that breakfast contributed to the higher proportion of daily calcium and milk - in its different forms - was the primary source of calcium in breakfast (69–74% across the age groups) [9].

In Denmark, breakfast commonly consumed foods include bread, breakfast cereals, and dairy products, as well as water, coffee, and juice, while intakes of fruits, vegetables, cakes, and soft drinks are low. These data were derived from a cross-sectional national food consumption study with a total of 3680 participants aged 6–75 years. In regards to the nutrient profile, researchers found that breakfast displayed relatively high amounts of dietary fiber, B vitamins, calcium and magnesium and low added sugar, total fat, sodium, vitamin A and D [10].

Gaal et al. (2018) investigated nutrient and food group intakes at breakfast and their relationship to overall diet quality in the United Kingdom. The data revealed that breakfast was particularly rich in B vitamins, vitamin D, calcium, iron, iodine, and magnesium. Tea, coffee, water, and semi-skimmed milk represented the foods with the highest percentage of consumers in all age groups. In regards to the energy intake contribution, "other" breakfast cereals, high-fiber breakfast cereals, white bread, and semi-skimmed milk stood out. In children and adolescents, high-fiber breakfast cereals, "other" breakfast cereals, semi-skimmed and whole milk, white bread, and reduced-fat spread were the main responsible for achieving micronutrient intake [11].

Most studies about the association between breakfast and health available in the literature were performed in the United States and Northern Europe. However, differences in breakfast may be identified among different cultures. The typical Italian breakfast, for example, includes milk, yogurt, coffee, tea, crispbread/rusks, breakfast cereals, brioche, biscuits, honey, sugar, and jam [12].

In a general way, the Western breakfast pattern is composed of bread, ready-to-eat cereal and/or milk. Additionally, many individuals are now opting for convenient liquid breakfast alternatives such as smoothies, which are blended beverages that typically contain fruit, yogurt, milk, honey, and fruit juice. A recent survey from Australia showed that ~32% of individuals reported consuming one or more smoothies per week [13].

It is important to emphasize that the habit of skipping breakfast or having a poor quality breakfast may impact on the nutritional status of individuals [7]. Many variables may compromise the habit of eating breakfast, among which lack of time, waking up late, and no breakfast prepared at home [3]. In regards to the quality of the meal, an adequate breakfast should contain dairy, cereals, and fruits [7]. Besides those food groups, other recommendations for a healthy breakfast include vegetables, protein sources, and low-fat spreads and oils [11].

Among foods commonly present at breakfast that have been associated with health, milk, and cereals represent the most relevant results [12]. In the Mediterranean diet, consuming an adequate breakfast is considered crucial, and this meal is also characterized by the presence of dairy products, cereals, fruit, and healthy fats [1].

Dairy products are important sources of high-quality protein, calcium, magnesium, zinc, riboflavin, vitamin E, vitamin A, folate, thiamin, niacin, vitamin B6, and vitamin B12. Thus, the elimination of cow's milk and other dairy items from the breakfast and overall diet may lead to nutritional deficiencies [14]. Cow's milk allergy, lactose intolerance, food restriction associated with religion and vegetarianism are possible explanations for excluding dairy products from the diet. Therefore, it is crucial to provide alternative nutritional and sensorial quality products to ensure adequate nutrient ingestion among these individuals.

HEALTH CONDITIONS ASSOCIATED WITH COW'S MILK

The ingestion of cow's milk has been associated with some adverse reactions that may occur at any period of life starting from birth. The nature of these adverse reactions includes "milk allergy" and "milk intolerance." Milk allergy is a hypersensitivity reaction initiated by specific immunologic mechanisms. On the other hand, milk intolerance derives from a specific enzyme deficiency, commonly lactose intolerance, attributable to beta-galactosidase (lactase) deficiency [15].

Allergy to cow's milk is not caused by the milk as a whole but to some specific parts (epitopes) of proteins which can bind specific IgE. Many different proteins compose cow's milk. Some of these proteins are considered significant allergens, some minor ones, and others have been rarely associated with clinical reactions. The key allergens of cow's milk are distributed among the whey and casein fractions. It should be noted that milk allergens of various mammalian species cross-react, especially cow's, sheep's and goat's milk protein. Besides the IgE mediated process, cow's milk allergy may also be cell-mediated or even involve both mechanisms (antibody-mediated and cell-mediated) [15, 16].

Food allergy is, in general, more often observed among children than adults. The estimated incidence of food allergy in toddlers is 5-8%, while in adults, it is 1-2%. Birth cohort studies found that the prevalence of cow's milk allergy during infancy ranged from 1.9% in a Finnish study, 2.16% in the Isle of Wight, 2.22% in a study from Denmark, 2.24% in the Netherlands, and up to 4.9% in Norway [15].

The clinical presentations of cow's milk allergy include gastrointestinal symptoms, urticaria, atopic dermatitis, eczema, respiratory symptoms, and anaphylaxis. Patients display gastrointestinal symptoms in 32 to 60% of cases, skin symptoms in 5 to 90%, and anaphylaxis in 0.8 to 9% of cases, which represents the most prominent health concern regarding food allergies [15].

The management of cow's milk allergy is based on the avoidance of milk proteins. For breastfed allergic children, it is recommended that mothers continue to breastfeed while avoiding dairy products. As a consequence of the dairy-free diet, health professionals should advise parents to use calcium supplements. For non-breastfed infants, there are formulas available as substitutes [15]. Other allergic individuals, including older children, adolescents, and adults, should exclude any milk-containing food from the diet and use alternative plant-based products [14]. In any case, suitable food substitutes must be under the national context and clinical setting of the individual, with adaptations to meet the patient's needs and values [15].

Lactose intolerance (LI), as opposed to cow's milk allergy, is not originated due to immune-mediated reactions elicited by proteins. LI may be described as a syndrome with different symptoms upon the consumption of lactose-containing food that derives from an insufficient level of the enzyme lactase in the brush border of the small bowel mucosa. Lactose is a disaccharide composed of galactose and glucose found in dairy products. As a consequence of the absence of the enzyme lactase, lactose is not correctly digested, and it can be fermented by gut microbiota, which explains LI symptoms such as abdominal pain, bloating, flatulence, and diarrhea. Individuals with LI may display different degrees of intolerance, depending on the severity of symptoms [17].

LI represents one of the most common forms of food intolerance [17], and four possible causes for its development have been described in the literature. The first form, which is rare, refers to Congenital Lactase Deficiency caused by recessive genetic mutations in the intestinal lactase enzyme. This form is associated with severe diarrhea acidosis and hypercalcemia, which appear rapidly with the beginning of breastfeeding. The second form - Developmental Lactase Deficiency - may be identified in premature neonates due to not fully established intestinal lactase production. Adult-onset hypolactasia is originated due to several polymorphisms in the transcription promoter region of the lactase gene and represents the main form of lactose maldigestion. At last, lactose maldigestion may present as a consequence of diseases that causes loss or injury to the small bowel, affecting lactase production - Secondary Lactase Deficiency [18].

Some strategies have been proposed to help controlling LI, such as the ingestion of lactose-free and lactose-reduced products and/or plant-based dairy substitutes and the use of prebiotics, exogenous oral lactase and probiotics [18]. The restriction of milk and milk-containing products may reduce or even eliminate LI manifestations. However, it is essential to emphasize that the individual experience following lactose ingestion depends on the amount of consumed lactose, type of food and food components in the meal, lactase concentration in the intestinal mucosa, and patient sensibility to symptoms [19].

DAIRY-FREE DIET AND MILK RESTRICTION

Factors such as cow's milk allergy, lactose intolerance, high cholesterol levels and an increasing number of adherents to vegetarian and vegan diets have pushed the population and the food industry to look up for alternatives to cow's milk [20].

Individuals who cannot consume cow's milk for any reason, whether it is a pathological or ideological reason, look for substitutes that are similar to cow's milk from a sensory and emotional point of view, while do not cause any discomfort after consumption [21]. Therefore, the food industry aims to create products that display similar appearance, taste, and nutritional composition of cow's milk [22].

Although some dairy-free products are already part of traditional cultures diets, there is a new interest of the population in these products, which are the plant-based milk and its derived products. The expanded plant-based food market is at an accelerated rate. Currently, the most popular ingredients used in the production of plant-based milk are soy, almonds, and rice [23]. However, plant-based milk based on hemp seeds, cashew, coconut, oats, macadamia, quinoa, peanuts, hazelnuts, and several other ingredients can also be found [20, 23].

It should be noted that the terms "milk," "cheese" and "yogurt" are associated with products originating from cow's milk. However, plant-based milk and their derivatives were labelled in the same way to reach the expectations of their consumers. There is a debate about whether these products can be called "milk," because its concept is defined as a whitish fluid liquid, rich in lipids and proteins produced by the mammary glands of mammalian animals [20]. However, throughout this chapter, the terms "milk," "cheese" and "yoghurt" were used for dairy-free products for a better understanding of the reader.

Plant-based milk are water-soluble extracts based on oilseeds, cereals, pseudocereals and/or legumes. The preparation depends on different steps, but the production flowchart is essentially the same: the raw material is previously soaked for a few hours and then processed with water. Then, the produced extract is filtered to remove insoluble residues. Other ingredients such as oils, flavorings, sugar, and stabilizers can be added to the final product. At the end of production, stability, homogenization, and pasteurization processes occur, generating colloidal suspensions or emulsions liquid extracts [23, 24].

Almond, cashew, coconut, hazelnut, oat, rice, and soy are the most common ingredients for plant-based milk production in the market [14].

These beverages generally resemble cow's milk in appearance, except for rice and oat extracts. However, the taste is not yet considered habitual to the western people. Damasceno, Botelho, and Alencar developed a chickpea and coconut beverage with 70% acceptance with the proportion of 70% chickpea and 30% coconut, showing improvements for taste among consumers. Besides, plant-based milk made with almonds, cashew, and hazelnuts, and with some legumes, such as soy and peanuts, are allergenic [25, 26].

Another issue that must be mentioned is the price of these products. Schuster et al. (2018) compared the price of a gallon for various plant-based milk and cow's milk and found that the cheapest gallon was cow's milk ($4.16/gallon), and the most expensive was coconut beverage ($10.14/gallon), and the average price of plant-based milk was around $6.85/gallon [27]. Thus, the high price of plant-based milk must be taken into account.

Another dairy food also widely consumed for breakfast is yogurt, and its substitutes are the plant-based yogurts. Plant-based yogurts represent an essential segment of dairy-free alternatives, with good demand among those individuals who need to replace cow's milk and dairy products [28].

Plant-based yogurt is prepared through the fermentation of the aqueous extract from different raw materials (legumes, seeds, cereals, and others). Among these raw materials used for the development of plant-based yogurts, soy and coconut stand out. Soy milk seems to be a good substrate to produce lactic acid bacteria commonly used in yogurt production [28].

The challenges faced by the food industry in the production of plant-based yogurts are associated with the appearance and texture of the final product. The phase separation that can occur in these products is the most common challenge. Therefore, a combination of gelling agents such as natural gums, proteins, starches, pectin, and agar are often used to provide a gel-type product with an acceptable texture and similar to dairy yogurt [28].

Another option in the dairy-free diet is tofu, known as vegan "cheese," which is prepared from soy curd, obtained by precipitation of soy milk proteins. Among the dairy-free alternatives, tofu becomes an exciting option, because it is a fermented product. Fermentation reduces the anti-nutritional factors found in soy, increasing the bioavailability of isoflavones, and promoting protein digestion. Besides, the fermentation process decreases the "beany" flavor intrinsic to soy [29].

From tofu, the food industry has also created different types of "cheeses," such as mozzarella and hard-type imitation cheese, varying the degree of ripeness and the ingredients and flavorings used [29].

Thus, the options for replacing cow's milk and dairy products nowadays are many. The market for these products grows every day, and it is increasingly common to find these products in markets, which expands the range of options for individuals who need to replace cow's milk in the diet.

BREAKFAST DAIRY-FREE ALTERNATIVES

Nutritional Aspects of Breakfast Dairy-Free Alternatives

The nutritional properties of plant-based milk will depend on the quality and type of the raw material, and also the type of processing [25]. Some of these beverages contain minimal amounts of protein, calcium, and iron when compared to cow's milk [14, 25]. Half of the samples analyzed in the study by Jeske et al. (2016) [23], among them plant-based milk based on rice, almonds, quinoa, and cashew nuts, contained less than 0.5% of proteins and only soy extract had values similar to cow's milk. In a study by Makinen et al. (2015) [24], a total of 3.32% of protein was found in cow's milk and 2.95% in soy extract. However, about 14% of patients who are allergic to cow's milk also show reactions to soy [21]. This allergenic characteristic of soy and peanuts was the motive for Damasceno, Botelho, and Alencar [26] to develop plant-based milk made from chickpea. The most accepted concentration reached 1.9% of protein, higher than the non-alergenic plant-based options in the market.

Therefore, the disadvantages of substituting cow's milk for plant-based milk are the low protein content and /or allergenicity of some of them [21]. However, it is entirely viable to have a dairy-free breakfast, as long as there is a balance in nutrient intake during the day, so it becomes healthier and complete. If the plant-based milk or yogurt contains low amounts of protein, for example, a solution could be the inclusion of foods that are a source of protein in the meal. Options are eggs (if the individual is not vegan) or even the addition of some isolated or hydrolyzed protein to the breakfast, such as pea and rice protein.

Regarding lipids content, the plant-based milk analyzed by Makinen at al. (2015) that obtained the highest lipid amount were cow's milk (3.5%) and quinoa extract (2.4%), while oat and rice extracts contained less than 1% of fat. Although these studied plant-based milk had low lipid content, their caloric value is similar to that of skimmed milk, energy coming mainly from carbohydrates [24].

The substitution of cow's milk for some plant-based milk must take into account that some nutrients, such as protein, calcium, iron, zinc, vitamin D, and B12 vitamin, are present in sufficient nutritional densities only in foods from animal sources. Thus, there must be compensation for nutrients from other foods when this substitution is made [22].

It is difficult to compare the nutritional profile of plant-based milk with cow's milk, as chemical composition data are often not available for some plant-based milk [14], such as information about potassium and sodium levels, for example.

Concerning calcium, a micronutrient related to bone health [22], the values are quite varied among plant-based milk. Chalupa-Krebzdak et al. (2018) found in their review study calcium values of 113 mg/100 g in soy extract, 58.67 mg/100 g in coconut extract, 118 mg/100 g in rice extract, 12 mg/100 g in hemp seeds extract, 160 mg/100 g in almond extract and 98.5 mg/100 g in cashew nut extract. Some of these commercial plant-based milk are fortified by the food industry to make them comparable to cow's milk, which has close to 113 mg/100 g of calcium [30]. Soy, almond, and rice extracts are generally enriched with calcium carbonate and/or tri-calcium phosphate by the food industry. Chickpea and coconut milk presented calcium content from 107.4 mg/100g to 131.3 mg/100g without fortification [26]. When cow's milk is replaced by unfortified plant-based milk, there is a risk of nutritional deficiencies, such as calcium, zinc, iodine, vitamins B2, B12, and D, especially if there is no consumption of animal source foods, as in vegan diets [22].

The nutritional composition of plant-based yogurt will depend on the type of raw material used for its preparation. In a study by Grasso, Alonso-Miravalles & O'Mahony (2020), the chemical composition of five types of commercial plant-based yogurt (soy, coconut, cashew, almonds, and hemp) and dairy yogurt was analyzed. They found a range from 0.6 to 4.6 g/100g of protein. The lowest values were observed for coconut and hemp-based yogurt (0.6g/100g) and the highest for soy yogurt (4.6 g/100g), which is the closest match to the protein values found in dairy yogurt (5.1 g/100g) [28].

Regarding the lipid content, the values ranged from 1.5 g/100g for dairy yogurt to 7.9 g/100g for almond yogurt. The high values for lipids in almond and coconut-based yogurts imply higher caloric values (79 and 97 Kcal, respectively) compared to the others (38 Kcal for hemp yogurt at 70 Kcal in cashew-based yogurt). Coconut yogurt had higher carbohydrate content (8 g/100g) and soy yogurt, the lower concentration of this macronutrient (1 g/100 g) [28].

According to data from the USDA database, the nutritional composition of tofu (100g) is approximately 82 Kcal with 10.6 g/100g of proteins, 2.3 g/100g of fats, and 3.5 g/100g of carbohydrates. In contrast, in 100 grams of mozzarella cheese, there is 295 Kcal with 24 g/100 g of proteins, 20 g/100 g of fats, and 5.6 g/100 g of carbohydrates [31]. That is, in nutritional terms, the values found in tofu and mozzarella cheese, for example, are quite different. Nevertheless, the nutritional composition of soy-based cheese, such as tofu, has been improved by the industry with the addition of soy flour, isolated soy protein, and hydrolyzed soy protein, as well as the development of probiotics cheese types [29].

Sensorial Aspects of Breakfast Dairy-Free Alternatives

When it comes to the overall acceptability of these products, an important limiting factor is consumers' unwillingness to try new foods. Despite this, soy milk - because it is already a traditional food on the market - has improved its sensory quality after several studies and attempts by the industry that was satisfactory in this regard. Taste is the essential criterion in the intention to purchase a product, and the information about good and/or familiar taste draws the consumer's attention. However, the presence of health benefits associated with the food also became an important criterion in the intention to purchase a product nowadays [24].

In general, plant-based milk have low acceptability by general consumers, who describe these beverages as having a chalky mouthfeel texture and legume-based milk as presenting a "beany" flavor. However, this "beany" flavor can be reduced using technological processes such as roasting and bleaching [32]. No other ingredient addition can justify the low scores observed in most studies of sensory analysis for plant-based milk. Sugar, coffee, or chocolate are common practice of cow's milk consumers, as well as plant-based milk consumers. Damasceno, Botelho, and Alencar [26] reached acceptability above 70% with consumers for chickpea and coconut beverage when the vanilla extract was added. An example of this can be noted in the study by Makinen et al. (2015), in which pure cow's milk was sensory evaluated, using a 9-point hedonic scale. The scores obtained for "odor" and "flavor" attributes were 5.2 and 5.79, respectively. Thus, even cow's milk did not reach acceptance scores when pure consumed [24].

Concerning the acceptability of plant-based yogurts, Grasso, Alonso-Miravalles & O'Mahony (2020) found in their study higher scores for the attribute "appearance" of dairy and coconut yogurt (7.17 and 6.93, respectively, on a scale of 1 to 10), and better scores for the attribute "odor" also for dairy and coconut yogurt (6.33 and 6.43, respectively). As for the "flavor," the best scores were obtained from soy and dairy yogurts (5.75 and 5.67, respectively). Regarding "texture," the yogurts with the highest scores were soy (6.49) and coconut (6.37). Soy and dairy yogurts received the highest scores for overall acceptability (5.75, both). The sensory analysis carried out in this study showed that coconut and soy-based yogurts are accepted and pleasant as much as dairy yogurt [28].

One of the barriers to the acceptability of soy-based products such as tofu is the "beany" flavor and its grainy texture, while dairy cheese has a smooth and uniform texture. These characteristics decrease the acceptance of soy-milk and soy-based products by consumers. However, the food industry has managed during the production of these "cheeses" by adding ingredients such as carrots to improve the color and flavor [29].

CONCLUSION

Breakfast constitutes an essential meal since it provides a considerable proportion of the daily nutrients intake. Moreover, the consumption of breakfast has been associated with better overall diet quality and reduced risk of health complications - such as weight gain and hypertension - when compared to breakfast skipping. It is noticeable that the breakfast nutritional profile may vary according to socioeconomic factors and individual and cultural habits, among others. However, a common feature between breakfasts worldwide is the presence of milk and dairy products at this meal.

Milk and other dairy products represent essential sources of high-quality protein, calcium, magnesium, and vitamin D. Therefore, the restriction of these foods from breakfast and the diet as a whole may contribute to lower ingestion of such nutrients. Cow's milk allergy, lactose intolerance, religious associated diet restrictions, and vegetarianism are some possible explanations for the absence or reduction of milk in the diet. As a consequence, the market for substitutes for dairy products has expanded in the last years, especially regarding the development of plant-based products. Nevertheless, nutritional and sensorial aspects of these products must be assessed to guarantee equal product quality for the consumers.

Regarding the nutritional composition of cow's milk substitutes, the beverage that most closely matches the composition of cow's milk is soy milk, although this is also an allergenic food. The other plant-based milk, such as almond, rice, and coconut extracts, are also good options, as long as they are combined with other protein source foods.

Despite the food industry efforts, alternative plant-based products are not yet wholly successful in the substitution of milk and dairy products. Although it is essential to provide alternatives for those who need, such as allergic individuals, it should be emphasized that the inappropriate dairy avoidance may negatively impact health, including substantial health implications for young children. Therefore, a proper evaluation of the need to avoid milk and dairy should be carried out before initiating restrictive diets.

REFERENCES

[1] Monteagudo, C.; Palacín-Arce, A.; Bibiloni, M. del M.; Pons, A.; Tur, J. A.; Olea-Serrano, F.; Mariscal-Arcas, M. Proposal for a Breakfast Quality Index (BQI) for children and adolescents. *Public Health Nutr.* 2012, *16*, 639–644, doi:10.1017/S1368980012003175.

[2] Matsumoto, M.; Hatamoto, Y.; Sakamoto, A.; Masumoto, A.; Ikemoto, S. Breakfast skipping is related to inadequacy of vitamin and mineral intakes among Japanese female junior high school students: a cross-sectional study. *J. Nutr. Sci.* 2020, doi:10.1017/jns.2019.44.

[3] Al-hazzaa, H. M.; Alhowikan, A. M.; Alhussain, M. H.; Obeid, O. A. *Breakfast consumption among Saudi primary-school children relative to sex and socio-demographic factors.* 2020, 1–14.

[4] Matthys, C.; Henauw, S. De; Bellemans, M.; Maeyer, M. De; Backer, G. De *Breakfast habits affect overall nutrient profiles in adolescents.* 2007, *10*, 413–421, doi:10.1017/S1368980007248049.

[5] Champilomati, G.; Notara, V.; Prapas, C.; Konstantinou, E.; Kordoni, M.; Velentza, A.; Mesimeri, M.; Antonogeorgos, G.; Rojas-gil, A. P.; Kornilaki, E. N.; Lagiou, A. *Breakfast consumption and obesity among preadolescents: An epidemiological study.* 2020, 81–88, doi:10.1111/ped.14050.

[6] Bellisle, F.; Vieux, F. *Breakfast Consumption in French Children, Adolescents, and Adults: A Nationally Representative Cross-Sectional Survey Examined in the Context of the International Breakfast Research Initiative.* 2018, doi:10.3390/nu10081056.

[7] Díaz-Torrente, X.; Quintiliano-Scarpelli, D. Dietary patterns of breakfast consumption among chilean university students. *Nutrients* 2020, *12*, doi:10.3390/nu12020552.

[8] de Sousa, J. R.; Botelho, R. B. A.; Akutsu, R. de C. C. A.; Zandonadi, R. P. Nutritional Quality of Breakfast Consumed by the Low-Income Population in Brazil: A Nationwide Cross-Sectional Survey. *Nutrients* 2019, *11*, 1418, doi:10.3390/nu11061418.

[9] Ruiz, E.; Ávila, J. M.; Valero, T.; Rodriguez, P.; Varela-Moreiras, G. Breakfast consumption in Spain: Patterns, nutrient intake and quality. findings from the ANIBES study, a study from the international breakfast research initiative. *Nutrients* 2018, *10*, doi:10.3390/nu10091324.

[10] Fagt, S.; Matthiessen, J.; Thyregod, C.; Kørup, K.; Biltoft-Jensen, A. Breakfast in Denmark. Prevalence of consumption, intake of foods, nutrients and dietary quality. a study from the international breakfast research initiative. *Nutrients* 2018, *10*, doi:10.3390/nu10081085.

[11] Gaal, S.; Kerr, M. A.; Ward, M.; McNulty, H.; Livingstone, M. B. E. Breakfast consumption in the UK: Patterns, nutrient intake and diet quality. a study from the international breakfast research initiative group. *Nutrients* 2018, *10*, doi:10.3390/nu10080999.

[12] di Giuseppe, R.; Di Castelnuovo, A.; Melegari, C.; De Lucia, F.; Santimone, I.; Sciarretta, A.; Barisciano, P.; Persichillo, M.; De Curtis, A.; Zito, F.; Krogh, V.; Donati, M. B. B.; de Gaetano, G.; Iacoviello, L.; Moli-sani Project Investigators Typical breakfast food consumption and risk factors for cardiovascular disease in a large sample of Italian adults. *Nutr. Metab. Cardiovasc. Dis.* 2012, *22*, 347–354, doi:10.1016/j.numecd.2010.07.006.

[13] Mccartney, D.; Langston, K.; Desbrow, B.; Khalesi, S. The influence of a fruit smoothie or cereal and milk breakfast on subsequent dietary intake : a pilot study. *Int. J. Food Sci. Nutr.* 2019, *0*, 1–11, doi:10.1080/09637486.2018.1547690.

[14] Singhal, S.; Baker, R. D.; Baker, S. S. A Comparison of the Nutritional Value of Cow's Milk and Nondairy Beverages. *JPGN* 2017, *64*, 799–805, doi:10.1097/MPG.0000000000001380.

[15] Fiocchi, A.; Brozek, J.; Schu, H.; Berg, A. Von; Beyer, K.; Bozzola, M.; Bradsher, J.; Compalati, E.; Ebisawa, M.; Guzman, M. A.; Li, H.; Heine, R. G.; Keith, P.; Lack, G.; Landi, M.; Martelli, A.; Rancé, F.;

Sampson, H.; Stein, A.; Terracciano, L.; Vieths, S.; Bradsher, J.; Allergy, F.; Network, A. World Allergy Organization (WAO) Diagnosis and Rationale for Action against Cow's Milk Allergy (DRACMA) Guidelines. *WAO J.* 2010, 57–161.

[16] Fiocchi, A.; Dahda, L.; Dupont, C.; Campoy, C.; Fierro, V.; Nieto, A. Cow ' s milk allergy: towards an update of DRACMA guidelines. *World Allergy Organ. J.* 2016, 1–11, doi:10.1186/s40413-016-0125-0.

[17] Costanzo, D. M.; Canani, R. B. Lactose Intolerance: Common Misunderstandings. *Ann. Nutr. Metab.* 2019, *73*, 30–37, doi:10.1159/000493669.

[18] Szilagyi, A.; Ishayek, N. *Lactose Intolerance, Dairy Avoidance, and Treatment Options.* 2018, doi:10.3390/nu10121994.

[19] Rosado, J. L. Intolerancia a la lactosa. 2016, 67–73.

[20] Vanga, S. K.; Raghavan, V. How well do plant based alternatives fare nutritionally compared to cow's milk? *J. Food Sci. Technol.* 2018, *55*, 10–20, doi:10.1007/s13197-017-2915-y.

[21] Jeske, S.; Zannini, E.; Arendt, E. K. Past, present and future: The strength of plant-based dairy substitutes based on gluten-free raw materials. *Food Res. Int.* 2018, *110*, 42–51, doi:10.1016/j.foodres.2017.03.045.

[22] Ahrens, K. E. S.; Ahrens, F.; Barth, C. A.; Barth, C. A. Nutritional and health attributes of milk and milk imitations. *Eur. J. Nutr.* 2019, *0*, 0, doi:10.1007/s00394-019-01936-3.

[23] Jeske, S.; Zannini, E.; Arendt, E. K. Evaluation of Physicochemical and Glycaemic Properties of Commercial Plant-Based Milk Substitutes. *Plant Foods Hum. Nutr.* 2017, *72*, 26–33, doi:10.1007/s11130-016-0583-0.

[24] Mäkinen, O. E.; Uniacke-Lowe, T.; O'Mahony, J. A.; Arendt, E. K. Physicochemical and acid gelation properties of commercial UHT-treated plant-based milk substitutes and lactose free bovine milk. *Food Chem.* 2015, *168*, 630–638, doi:10.1016/j.foodchem.2014.07.036.

[25] Mäkinen, O. E.; Wanhalinna, V.; Zannini, E.; Arendt, E. K. Foods for Special Dietary Needs: Non-Dairy Plant Based Milk Substitutes and

Fermented Dairy Type Products. *Crit. Rev. Food Sci. Nutr.* 2016, *56*, 339–349, doi:10.1080/10408398.2012.761950.

[26] Arruda Daguer Damasceno, L. R.; Assunção Botelho, R. B.; Rodrigues de Alencar, E. Development of novel plant-based milk based on chickpea and coconut. *LWT* 2020, 109479, doi:10.1016/j.lwt.2020.109479.

[27] Schuster, M. J.; Wang, X.; Hawkins, T.; Painter, J. E. Comparison of the Nutrient Content of Cow's Milk and Nondairy Milk Alternatives. *Nutr. Today* 2018, *53*, 153–159, doi:10.1097/NT.0000000000000284.

[28] Grasso, N.; Alonso-miravalles, L.; Mahony, J. A. O. Composition, Physicochemical and Sensorial Properties of Commercial Plant-Based Yogurts. 2020, doi:10.3390/foods9030252.

[29] Jeewanthi, R. K. C.; Paik, H.-D. Modifications of nutritional, structural, and sensory characteristics of non-dairy soy cheese analogs to improve their quality attributes. *J. Food Sci. Technol.* 2018, *55*, 4384–4394, doi:10.1007/s13197-018-3408-3.

[30] Chalupa-krebzdak, S.; Long, C. J.; Bohrer, B. M. Nutrient density and nutritional value of milk and plant-based milk alternatives. *Int. Dairy J.* 2018, doi:10.1016/j.idairyj.2018.07.018.

[31] USDA Food Data Central Database.

[32] Silva, A. R. A.; Silva, M. M. N.; Ribeiro, B. D. Health Issues and Technological Aspects of Plant-based Alternative Milk. *Food Res. Int.* 2019, 108972, doi:10.1016/j.foodres.2019.108972.

INDEX

A

academic performance, 105
acceptability, 52, 115, 116
adolescents, 2, 6, 8, 11, 12, 14, 74, 92, 104, 105, 106, 107, 109, 118
adult education, 87
allergens, 91, 108
allergic reaction, 90
allergy, ix, x, 11, 40, 59, 61, 85, 92, 104, 108, 109, 110, 117, 120
almonds, 111, 112, 113, 115
anaphylaxis, 92, 109
animal-based meals, viii, 33
ataxia, ix, 59, 61, 85, 92
atherosclerosis, 35
atopic dermatitis, 109
avoidance, 43, 109, 117

B

beef, 7, 38, 45, 71
benefits, viii, 1, 3, 15, 33, 35, 41, 42, 43, 46, 66, 67, 71, 79, 116
beverages, viii, 33, 39, 40, 46, 107, 112, 113, 116
bicarbonate, 69
bioavailability, 12, 13, 66, 112
blood, 10, 13, 36, 37
blood pressure, 13
body fat, 10, 36, 38
body weight, 37
Brazil, ix, 1, 5, 6, 7, 11, 17, 20, 24, 28, 30, 31, 33, 59, 63, 71, 74, 76, 83, 84, 85, 92, 94, 95, 96, 103, 119
Brazilian public schools, v, vii, ix, 83, 84, 85
breakfast, v, vi, vii, viii, ix, x, 1, 2, 3, 5, 6, 7, 9, 17, 18, 19, 20, 21, 22, 23, 24, 25, 26, 27, 28, 29, 30, 31, 32, 33, 34, 35, 38, 39, 40, 41, 42, 43, 44, 45, 46, 47, 48, 50, 52, 54, 55, 56, 59, 60, 62, 63, 66, 67, 69, 70, 71, 76, 84, 94, 95, 96, 103, 104, 105, 106, 107, 108, 112, 113, 115, 117, 118, 119
breakfast cereals, 38, 42, 46, 66, 67, 105, 106, 107
breastfeeding, 110

C

calcium, x, 3, 8, 9, 10, 11, 12, 13, 41, 45, 46, 88, 96, 104, 105, 106, 107, 108, 109, 113, 114, 117
calcium carbonate, 114
caloric intake, 4, 34, 46
cancer, 10, 13, 36, 41, 42
carbohydrates, viii, 8, 33, 38, 42, 43, 46, 64, 65, 69, 79, 95, 114, 115
cardiovascular disease, 10, 13, 15, 36, 37, 42, 104, 119
cardiovascular risk, 2, 37
celiac disease, vii, ix, x, 59, 61, 72, 74, 75, 84, 85, 89, 92, 93, 97, 98, 99, 102
cereal-grains, 60
cheese, viii, x, 5, 7, 33, 39, 42, 43, 45, 69, 71, 96, 104, 105, 111, 112, 113, 115, 116, 121
children, vii, ix, 2, 6, 8, 11, 12, 74, 75, 83, 84, 85, 86, 88, 89, 90, 92, 94, 95, 96, 105, 106, 107, 109, 118
chronic diseases, 36, 38, 42, 43, 44, 46
chronic kidney disease, 36
circadian rhythm, 34
coffee, viii, x, 5, 7, 11, 12, 13, 33, 39, 40, 42, 43, 95, 103, 106, 107, 116
cognitive development, 84, 89, 90, 96
cognitive function, 2
cognitive performance, 16
commercial, 69, 72, 79, 80, 114, 115, 120
composition, viii, 1, 2, 3, 7, 13, 24, 38, 41, 45, 52, 65, 66, 69, 78, 90, 111, 114, 115, 117, 121
consensus, 3, 16, 74
consumers, 3, 6, 11, 40, 41, 45, 64, 72, 105, 106, 107, 111, 112, 115, 116, 117
consumption, viii, ix, 1, 2, 3, 4, 5, 6, 7, 8, 9, 10, 11, 12, 13, 14, 15, 16, 34, 35, 36, 37, 38, 39, 40, 44, 46, 59, 60, 62, 63, 72, 76, 104, 105, 106, 109, 111, 114, 117, 118, 119
consumption patterns, 104, 105
contamination, ix, 60, 67, 72, 75, 80, 84, 85, 90, 91, 93, 96
cooking, 63, 68, 69, 81
cost, ix, 60, 62, 75, 91, 93, 94
cross-sectional study, 41, 118
cultural differences, 3
cultural influence, 7
culture, 5, 87, 88, 94, 96

D

dairy substitutes, 40, 110, 120
dairy-free products, 104, 111
Department of Agriculture, 43, 56
diet, vii, viii, ix, x, 4, 7, 8, 10, 11, 12, 14, 15, 16, 33, 35, 36, 37, 38, 40, 41, 43, 45, 59, 61, 62, 66, 72, 73, 84, 85, 89, 90, 91, 92, 93, 96, 104, 105, 106, 107, 108, 109, 112, 113, 117, 119
dietary fiber, 5, 64, 68, 107
dietary habits, 36
dietary intake, 119
digestibility, 66, 67, 77, 78, 79, 81
digestion, 64, 65, 78, 79, 113
diseases, viii, 3, 10, 15, 34, 36, 37, 44, 85, 90, 110
diversity, 2, 9, 70, 84
dough, 63, 67, 68, 69, 78

E

education, 87, 88, 90
emulsions, 111
energy, viii, 1, 2, 3, 4, 5, 7, 8, 9, 15, 16, 104, 105, 106, 107, 114
energy consumption, 3, 4, 15
energy density, 5
environmental contamination, 91

enzyme, 108, 109, 110
evidence, 3, 10, 13, 42, 61
exclusion, 36, 61, 64, 85, 91, 92

F

fat, 2, 5, 10, 15, 16, 38, 40, 42, 43, 65, 69, 89, 95, 104, 105, 107, 108, 114
fat intake, 40
fermentation, 63, 76, 112, 113
fiber, viii, 10, 34, 36, 38, 40, 44, 45, 64, 65, 67, 69, 70, 107
fibers, 3, 11, 44, 45, 46, 65, 67, 88
financial resources, 86, 87
fish, 5, 16, 35, 36, 39, 40, 71
flour, 39, 60, 63, 64, 65, 67, 68, 72, 78, 79, 81, 86, 93, 95, 96, 115
food, viii, ix, x, 2, 3, 4, 5, 6, 7, 8, 9, 10, 11, 13, 15, 16, 33, 35, 36, 38, 43, 44, 46, 60, 61, 62, 63, 64, 67, 69, 70, 71, 75, 77, 79, 83, 84, 85, 86, 87, 88, 89, 90, 91, 92, 93, 94, 95, 96, 103, 104, 105, 106, 107, 108, 109, 110, 111, 112, 113, 114, 115, 116, 117, 119
food additive, 46
food choices, viii, 2, 16, 23, 35, 46
food habits, 94, 96, 105
food industry, x, 15, 16, 62, 64, 71, 104, 110, 111, 112, 113, 114, 117
food intake, viii, 13, 33, 44, 90
food production, 91
food products, 62
food safety, 91
food security, 89
food services, 62, 75
fruits, vii, viii, x, 2, 3, 5, 6, 7, 8, 9, 10, 11, 16, 34, 36, 38, 39, 43, 45, 62, 89, 95, 103, 105, 106, 107

G

glucose, 10, 34, 37, 42, 77, 109
gluten, v, vii, ix, 59, 60, 61, 62, 63, 64, 65, 66, 67, 68, 69, 70, 71, 72, 73, 74, 75, 77, 78, 79, 80, 81, 83, 84, 85, 86, 90, 91, 92, 93, 94, 95, 96, 99, 100, 101, 102, 120
gluten ataxia, ix, 59, 61, 85, 92
gluten-containing foods, ix, 59, 83, 85
gluten-free, v, ix, 59, 60, 61, 62, 66, 67, 68, 69, 70, 71, 72, 73, 74, 75, 77, 78, 79, 80, 81, 83, 84, 85, 90, 91, 92, 93, 94, 95, 96, 99, 100, 102, 120
gluten-free breakfast, v, 62, 66, 67, 80, 83, 95
gluten-free diet, ix, 59, 61, 62, 66, 73, 75, 84, 90, 92, 93, 96, 99, 102
gluten-related disorders, v, vii, ix, 59, 60, 73, 74, 83, 84, 85, 90, 92, 101
growth, 12, 15, 36, 60, 63, 66, 104
guidelines, 40, 87, 90, 91, 120

H

harmful effects, vii, ix, 15, 34
health, viii, 2, 3, 12, 15, 16, 32, 33, 34, 35, 36, 37, 41, 42, 43, 44, 46, 47, 66, 67, 71, 75, 79, 84, 88, 89, 90, 94, 96, 107, 108, 109, 114, 116, 117, 120
heart disease, 16, 34, 36
hemoglobin, 37, 42
high blood pressure, 10, 13
human, 3, 10, 15, 16, 79, 89, 94
human body, 10
human health, 15, 16
human right, 89, 94
hypertension, 89, 104, 117

I

individuals, vii, ix, x, 3, 4, 6, 13, 14, 34, 35, 40, 44, 60, 61, 67, 68, 72, 83, 85, 88, 89, 92, 104, 106, 107, 108, 109, 112, 113, 117
industry, 40, 60, 73, 75, 77, 114, 115
inflammation, 36, 38, 43, 44
inflammatory disease, 15
ingestion, 104, 106, 108, 110, 117
ingredients, x, 40, 41, 44, 45, 47, 61, 64, 66, 68, 69, 70, 71, 72, 81, 88, 90, 96, 104, 111, 113, 117
insulin, 10, 34, 37, 38, 43, 104
insulin resistance, 37
insulin sensitivity, 37, 38
inulin-type fructan, 64, 78
iodine, 41, 105, 107, 114
iron, 5, 8, 38, 45, 88, 96, 105, 107, 113, 114

L

lactase, 108, 109, 110
lactose, x, 11, 40, 89, 96, 104, 108, 109, 110, 117, 120
lactose intolerance, x, 11, 40, 89, 96, 98, 104, 108, 109, 110, 117, 120
lactose-free, 110
learning process, 87
legumes, 16, 36, 38, 40, 44, 45, 46, 50, 69, 71, 111, 112
lipids, 111, 114, 115
low-grade inflammation, 36, 37

M

magnesium, 5, 8, 45, 88, 105, 107, 108, 117
meat, 9, 15, 16, 35, 36, 39, 41, 71, 93
mechanical properties, 78
mental development, 105
meta-analysis, 9, 14, 35
metabolic dysfunction, 34
metabolism, 7, 10, 12, 34, 42
microbiota, 44, 109
micronutrients, 6, 9, 64, 88, 104
microorganisms, 66
microstructure, 77
milk allergy, x, 11, 104, 108, 109, 110, 117, 120
milk intolerance, 108
milk-free, x, 104
milk-free diet, x, 104
mortality, viii, 13, 34, 42, 43, 44
mucosa, 61, 109, 110
muscle contraction, 10

N

non-celiac gluten sensitive, 61
non-processed plant-based foods, 47
nutrients, 2, 3, 8, 10, 13, 16, 18, 20, 21, 22, 23, 28, 30, 41, 44, 45, 46, 49, 50, 52, 54, 55, 56, 66, 73, 74, 75, 76, 80, 81, 94, 95, 96, 99, 104, 105, 114, 117, 118, 119
nutrition, 8, 15, 34, 40, 75, 79, 87
nutritional deficiencies, 108, 114
nutritional status, viii, 2, 9, 107

O

obesity, viii, 1, 5, 6, 9, 10, 11, 15, 16, 42, 104, 118
osteoporosis, 10, 12
overweight, viii, ix, 1, 6, 10, 34
ovo-lacto-vegetarian diet, 40
oxidative stress, 37

P

participants, 6, 8, 9, 40, 41, 105, 106, 107

plant-based, v, viii, 11, 17, 30, 33, 34, 40, 41, 44, 45, 46, 47, 51, 52, 53, 54, 56, 104, 109, 110, 111, 112, 113, 114, 115, 116, 117, 120, 121
plant-based meal, viii, 33, 34
plant-based milk, 11, 17, 30, 40, 41, 45, 46, 52, 104, 111, 112, 113, 114, 116, 117, 120, 121
plant-based yogurt, 112, 115, 116, 121
population, ix, x, 5, 13, 14, 35, 40, 59, 61, 66, 87, 94, 95, 96, 104, 106, 110, 111
potassium, 8, 45, 105, 114
potato, 7, 64, 66, 68, 78, 93
potato starch, 64, 66, 93
potential benefits, 43, 47
preparation, iv, 16, 90, 96, 111, 115
prevention, vii, ix, 34, 44, 90
probiotics, 79, 110, 115
professionals, viii, 33, 42, 109
protein structure, 64
proteins, 3, 11, 38, 60, 69, 95, 108, 109, 111, 112, 113, 115
public schools, vii, ix, 11, 83, 84, 85, 94, 95

R

raw materials, 112, 120
reactions, ix, 59, 66, 108, 109, 113
recommendations, iv, viii, ix, 8, 15, 33, 35, 40, 43, 59, 62, 91, 108
researchers, 7, 16, 64, 71, 107
response, 10, 35, 43, 77, 78, 79, 92
restrictions, ix, 45, 83, 84, 89, 90, 96, 117
risk, viii, 1, 6, 9, 10, 12, 13, 34, 35, 36, 37, 38, 41, 42, 43, 44, 76, 85, 92, 96, 114, 117, 119
risk factors, 119

S

saturated fat, viii, 6, 14, 34, 36, 38, 41, 42, 43, 89
school, ix, 83, 84, 85, 86, 87, 88, 89, 90, 91, 93, 94, 95, 96, 105, 118
school meal, 84, 85, 86, 87, 88, 90, 94, 96, 100, 101, 102
school performance, 105
showing, 3, 16, 34, 42, 69, 112
social exclusion, 89
social movements, 85
social participation, 87
sodium, 2, 6, 8, 13, 14, 16, 40, 46, 68, 69, 89, 107, 114
soy-based, 6, 45, 115, 116
substitutes, ix, 40, 41, 45, 46, 60, 64, 83, 85, 93, 96, 109, 110, 111, 112, 117, 120

T

texture, 63, 67, 70, 79, 88, 95, 112, 116
tofu, 5, 71, 112, 113, 115, 116
treatment, 5, 37, 61, 62, 85, 92, 93
type 2 diabetes, 10, 34, 35, 37, 38, 42, 76, 104

V

vegan, 11, 34, 36, 37, 46, 49, 52, 110, 112, 114
vegetables, vii, viii, 3, 5, 7, 8, 10, 34, 36, 39, 43, 44, 45, 46, 71, 86, 89, 105, 106, 108
vegetarian, x, 25, 34, 35, 36, 37, 38, 40, 45, 46, 47, 48, 49, 50, 51, 52, 53, 55, 57, 104, 110
vegetarian diet, 25, 35, 36, 37, 38, 45, 46, 47, 48, 49, 50, 51, 52, 53, 55, 57
vegetarianism, 35, 36, 108, 117
vitamin A, 8, 107, 108

vitamin B1, 105, 108
vitamin B12, 108
vitamin B2, 105
vitamin B6, 108
vitamin C, 105
vitamin D, 12, 107, 114, 117
vitamin E, 108
vitamins, 3, 5, 8, 11, 41, 45, 62, 88, 105, 107, 114

W

water, 7, 45, 60, 63, 64, 67, 68, 69, 78, 81, 105, 106, 107, 111
weight control, 36, 37, 38, 62
weight gain, viii, 1, 34, 42, 104, 117
weight loss, 9, 34, 38, 43
wheat allergy, ix, 59, 61, 85, 92
whole-foods, ix, 34
worldwide, ix, x, 9, 13, 40, 59, 60, 71, 103, 105, 117